Exercise-Induced Acute Renal Failure

Acute Renal Failure with Severe Loin Pain and Patchy Renal Ischemia After Anaerobic Exercise

Isao Ishikawa

Exercise-Induced Acute Renal Failure

Acute Renal Failure with Severe Loin Pain and Patchy Renal Ischemia After Anaerobic Exercise

With 76 Figures, Including 5 in Color

Springer

Isao Ishikawa, M.D.
Emeritus Professor, Kanazawa Medical University
1-35 Kohyo-Dai, Uchinada, Kahoku, Ishikawa 920-0272, Japan;
Division of Nephrology, Asanogawa General Hospital
83 Kosaka-Naka, Kanazawa, Ishikawa 920-8621, Japan

Library of Congress Control Number: 2007926814

ISBN 978-4-431-69483-0 Springer Tokyo Berlin Heidelberg New York

Springer is a part of Springer Science+Business Media
springer.com

Printed in Japan

Typesetting: SNP Best-set Typesetter Ltd., Hong Kong
Printing and binding: Hicom, Japan

Printed on acid-free paper

Preface

There are two types of exercise-related acute renal failure, one of which is myoglobinuric acute renal failure. In myoglobinuric acute renal failure, strenuous exercise such as marathon running or mountain climbing causes marked rhabdomyolysis, resulting in myoglobinuria. However, Acute renal failure with severe Loin pain and Patchy renal ischemia after anaerobic Exercise (ALPE), which we describe in this text, differs from myoglobinuric acute renal failure. The first patient known to have ALPE attended an emergency outpatient unit one night with severe loin pain. Under a tentative diagnosis of ureteral stone, the patient underwent intravenous pyelography (IVP). However, there was no ureteral stone. Several hours later, a plain computed tomography (CT) scan revealed wedge-shaped contrast enhancement in the kidney. In 1981, we initially reported this finding as "patchy renal vasoconstriction in man" [1]. Thereafter, we encountered several patients with acute renal failure and some common characteristics. These were severe loin pain after exercise and wedge-shaped contrast enhancement in the kidney on CT, but with no marked increases in serum creatine phosphokinase (CPK)/myoglobin levels, as described for the first patient. In 1982, we reported this condition as a new acute renal failure syndrome [2]. A subsequent study showed that this type of acute renal failure frequently developed in patients with renal hypouricemia [3]. As this disorder is associated with anaerobic exercise, it is called acute renal failure with severe loin pain and patchy renal ischemia after anaerobic exercise (ALPE) [4].

In this text, we emphasize that ALPE should always be considered in patients who complain of severe loin pain and nausea after sprinting in an athletics meeting, and while ALPE frequently develops in patients with renal hypouricemia, it also develops in those without it.

We would like specialists in emergency care, general practitioners, nephrologists, pediatricians, school physicians, and sports physicians to read this text.

Contents

Color Plates

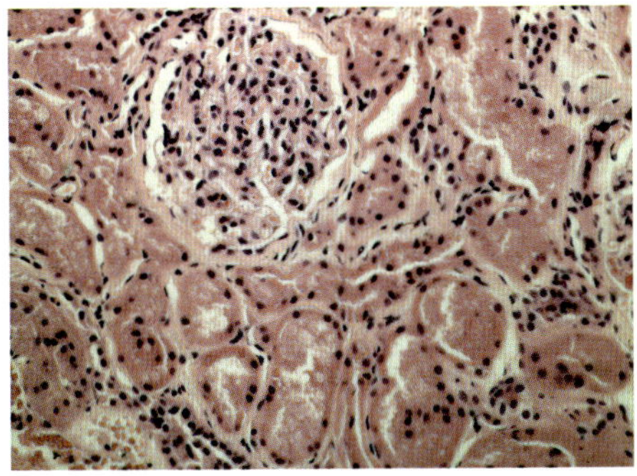

FIG. 4. Kidney biopsy. The findings suggested acute tubular necrosis (p. 4)

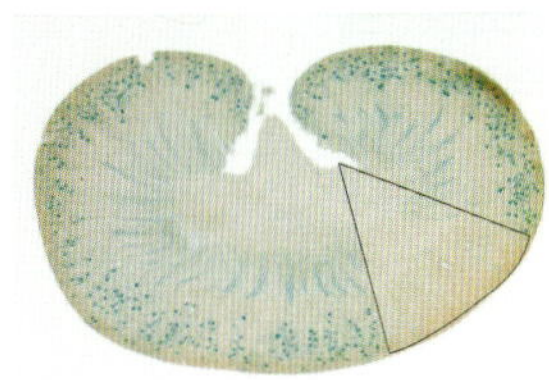

FIG. 5. The reason why we considered that wedge-shaped contrast enhancement reflected a vascular lesion. We infused microspheres in the rat heart, and performed glomerular supervital staining with Alcian blue. In this rat, renal infarction was detected. This was the basis of the hypothesis that wedge-shaped lesions are related to vasoconstriction (p. 4)

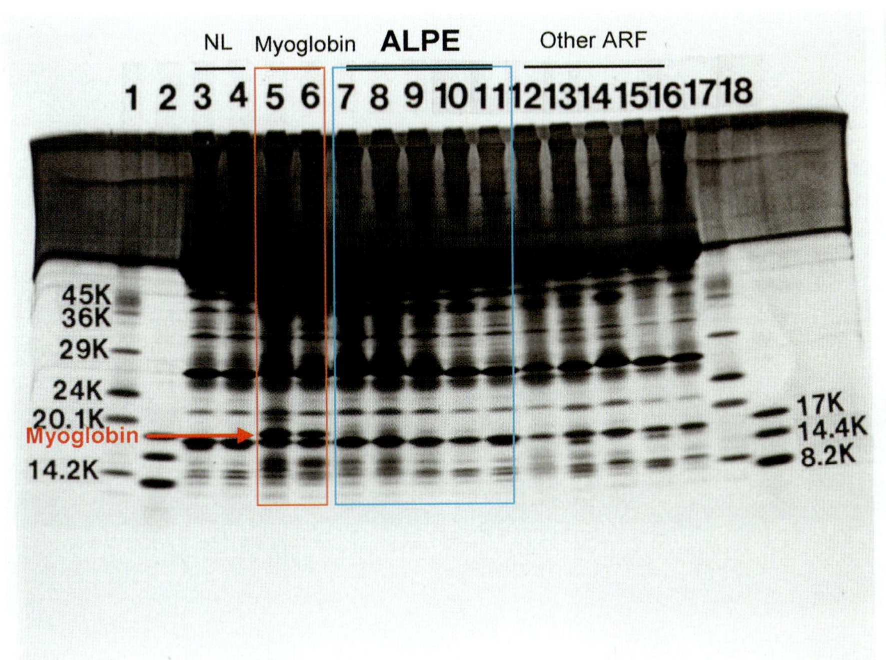

FIG. 62. SDS-PAGE in normal controls and in patients with myoglobinuric acute renal failure, ALPE, or acute renal failure related to other etiologies. There were no bands which were specific to ALPE. *ARF*, acute renal failure (p. 68)

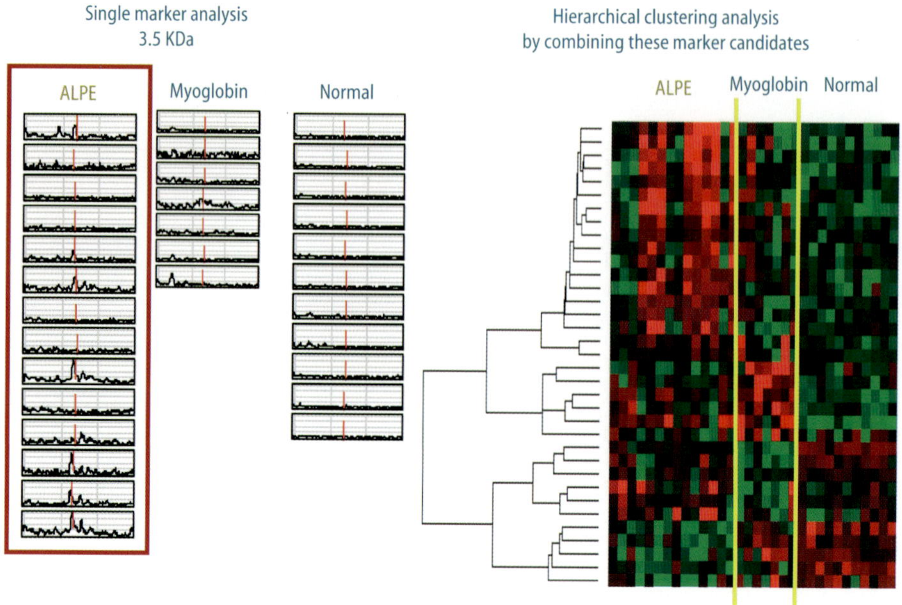

FIG. 64. Proteomic analysis with a SELDI–TOF–MS. In single marker analysis (*left*), the relative intensity of the 3.5 KDa peptide was high in the ALPE group. In the hierarchical clustering analysis with marker candidates, the heat map in the ALPE group differed from those in the myoglobinuric acute renal failure and normal groups (p. 69)

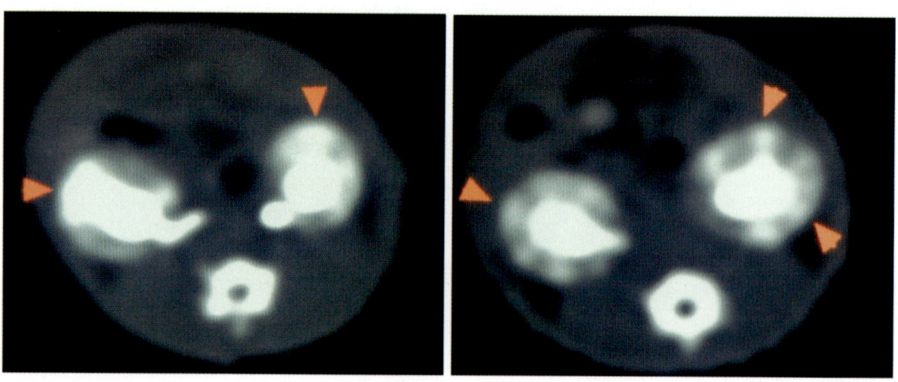

FIG. 72. Wedge-shaped contrast enhancement after the administration of vasopressin in an animal model (p. 73)

Chapter 1
Exercise-Related Acute Renal Failure

1 Description of Exercise-Related Acute Renal Failure

In 1910, Meyer-Betz reported the first published case of acute renal failure with muscular pain, weakness, and dark urine after intense exercise [5]. In 1960, Howenstine reported that this type of acute renal failure was exercise-related myoglobinuria [6]. However, at this time, it was impossible to distinguish hemoglobin from myoglobin, and this type of acute renal failure was considered to be a type of heat stroke. However, in 1970, Jackson [7] reported that this disorder was exercise-related renal failure and muscle damage, and this publication led to a gradual increase in research interest in myoglobinuric acute renal failure. In 1972, Hamilton et al. [8] and Knochel [9], respectively, reported that similar cases were exertional rhabdomyolysis. Matsumoto et al.[10] first reported this disorder in Japan in 1976.

In all case reports, the levels of creatine phosphokinase (CPK) were markedly increased to about 70 000 mU/ml or more [11]. Furthermore, this disorder frequently develops in people who are not accustomed to exercise, and is therefore called white-collar rhabdomyolysis [12], which indicates myoglobin-related acute renal failure.

In 1982, we classified exercise-related acute renal failure into two types: myoglobinuric acute renal failure, as had previously been reported, and non-myoglobin-related acute renal failure (exercise-induced acute renal failure). In 2002, the latter was named ALPE (Acute renal failure with severe Loin pain and Patchy renal ischemia after anaerobic Exercise) [4]. The term 'acute kidney injury' (AKI) has recently been proposed as a patho-physiologically more correct alternative to the term acute renal failure. Therefore, exercise-induced acute renal failure in this book may be replaced by exercise-induced acute kidney injury.

2 Myoglobinuric/Non-Myoglobinuric Acute Renal Failure

Exercise-related acute renal failure is classified into two types (Table 1). One type is myoglobinuric acute renal failure, in which strenuous exercise over a long period of time, such as marathon running and mountain climbing, causes severe rhabdomyolysis with myoglobinuria. The clinical course of myoglobinuric acute renal failure in one of our patients is shown in Fig. 1. The patient was a male student who developed this disorder during a Shorinji Kenpo (one of the combative sports with technique of bare hand self defense) training camp. His CPK level had increased to approximately 30 000 mU/ml, and dark urine and muscular pain in the upper and lower limbs were

TABLE 1. Exercise-related acute renal failure

Massive rhabdomyolysis—myoglobinuric acute renal failure due to marathon, mountain climbing, etc.
Minimum rhabdomyolysis—non-myoglobinuric acute renal failure due to exercise-induced acute renal failure—ALPE (acute renal failure with severe loin pain and patchy renal ischemia after anaerobic exercise) after sprint, short track event such as 200-m race, etc.

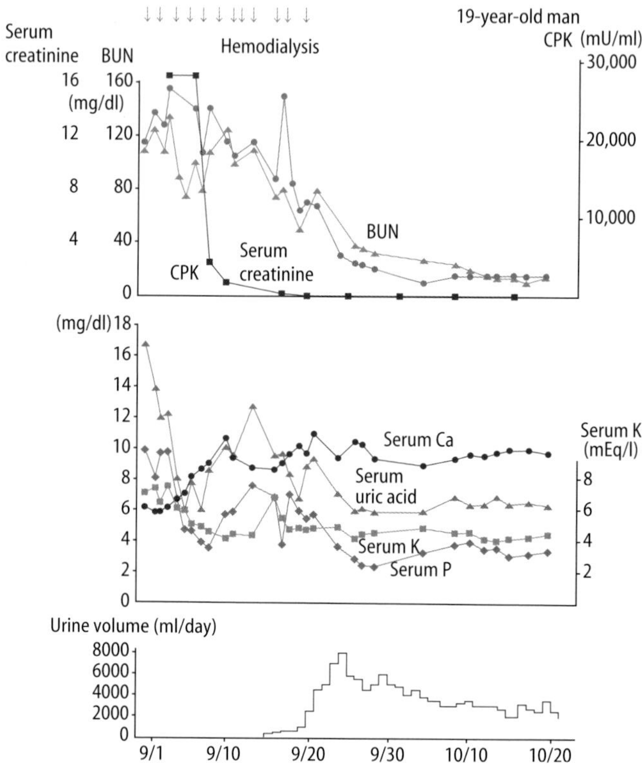

FIG. 1. Acute tubular necrosis (acute renal failure) due to myoglobinuria (rhabdomyolysis) after Shorinji Kenpo

noted. Furthermore, this patient showed a typical electrolyte imbalance in the presence of rhabdomyolysis, and required hemodialysis because of oliguria. This case is typical of exercise-related myoglobinuric acute renal failure.

The other type is non-myoglobinuric acute renal failure, in which intense exercise over a short period of time, such as sprinting, causes minimal rhabdomyolysis without myoglobinuria, i.e., acute renal failure syndrome with severe loin pain and patchy renal vasoconstriction [2]. A recent study showed that anaerobic exercise caused this syndrome, and proposed that "Acute renal failure with severe Loin pain and Patchy renal ischemia after anaerobic Exercise (ALPE) (exercise-induced acute renal failure)" was a new type of acute renal failure syndrome [4].

Chapter 2
Exercise-Induced Acute Renal Failure (ALPE)

1 The First Patient in Whom Wedge-Shaped Patchy Renal Ischemia was Demonstrated

The first patient to be recognized as having this condition was a 29-year-old man [1]. On August 20, 1979, he attended an emergency outpatient unit at night with severe loin pain. His serum creatinine level was slightly increased (1.6 mg/dl). Under a tentative diagnosis of ureteral stone, an intravenous pyelography (IVP) was performed. However, there was no stone. Plain computed tomography (CT) 22 h after the administration of a contrast medium (delayed CT: plain CT several hours or days after the administration of a contrast medium) (Fig. 2) showed patchy wedge-shaped contrast enhancement in the bilateral kidneys (the first image in a human). This persisted for 48 h after administration of the medium (Fig. 3) [1]. A kidney biopsy 2 weeks after onset suggested acute tubular necrosis (Fig. 4). At the same time, we were conducting an experiment involving an infusion of microspheres into a rat heart and glomerular supervital staining with Alcian blue, and we found some wedge-shaped lesions. As this finding suggested renal infarction (Fig. 5), we speculated that the wedge-shaped contrast enhancement in our patient was associated with a vascular lesion (vasoconstriction).

This case report was published in *Nephron* in 1981 as evidence for patchy renal vasoconstriction in humans [1].

2 Our Series in the Initial Phase

A 28-year-old man (Patient 1). This patient complained of a mild headache which persisted for 2 days, and took a mixed preparation consisting of aminopyrine at 108 mg and phenacetin at 400 mg at 0900 hours on October 14, 1979. After 1 h, he ran a 200-m race in an athletics meeting. Bilateral loin pain then occurred. After 8 h, the pain became severe and he attended an emergency outpatient unit during the night. Two days after onset, his serum creatinine level was 2.8 mg/dl, his serum myoglobin level was normal, and his creatine phosphokinase (CPK) level was slightly increased. Three days after onset, a new type of acute renal failure was suspected, and a CT scan of his kidneys was performed 2, 24, 48, and 72 h after the intravenous administration

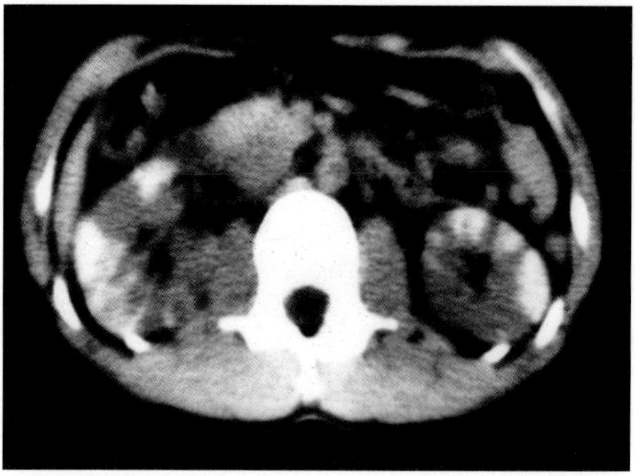

FIG. 2. Plain computed tomography (CT) 22 h after the administration of contrast medium. Wedge-shaped contrast enhancement was observed in the bilateral kidneys (From [1], with permission)

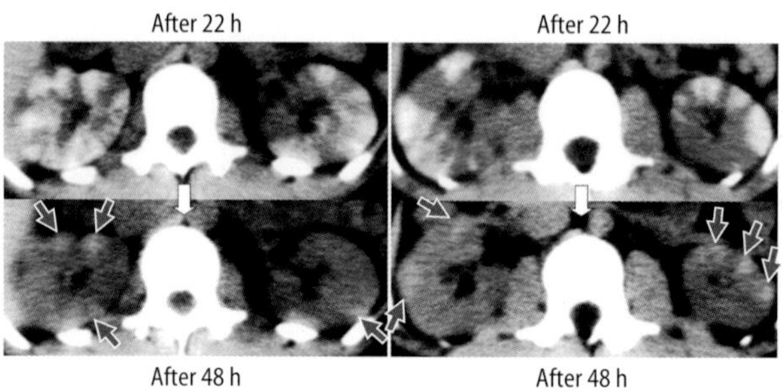

FIG. 3. Slight wedge-shaped contrast enhancement (*arrows*) was observed 48 h after the administration of contrast medium (*bottom*)

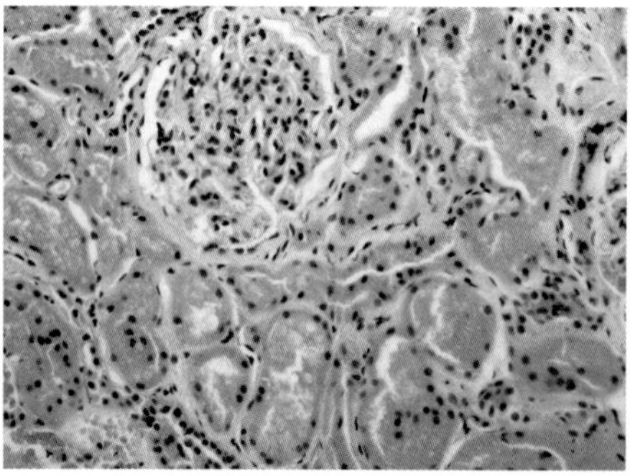

FIG. 4. Kidney biopsy. The findings suggested acute tubular necrosis

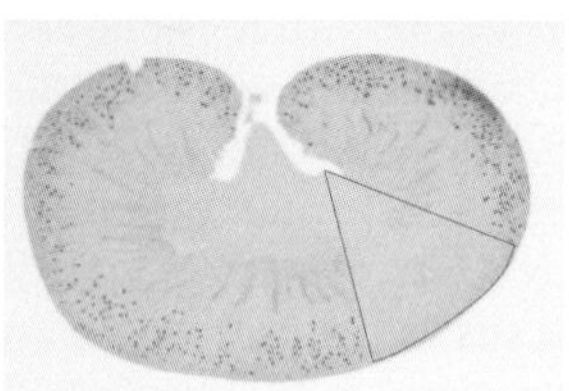

FIG. 5. The reason why we considered that wedge-shaped contrast enhancement reflected a vascular lesion. We infused microspheres in the rat heart, and performed glomerular supervital staining with Alcian blue. In this rat, renal infarction was detected. This was the basis of the hypothesis that wedge-shaped lesions are related to vasoconstriction

of a contrast medium (40 ml of 67% sodium iothalamate). The CT scan 48 h after administration of the medium (Fig. 6) showed diffuse to patchy contrast enhancement, and this finding persisted until 72 h after the contrast administration. The patient's serum creatinine level was 7.1 mg/dl 4 days after onset. However, oliguria was not observed, and conservative therapy reduced the level of serum creatinine. A kidney biopsy 36 days after onset suggested the regeneration of acute tubular necrosis. The loin pain persisted for 4 days.

A 24-year-old man (Patient 2). This patient participated in a 200-m swimming race at 1600 hours on August 9, 1980. Immediately after this exercise, headache and nausea developed. On August 10, severe bilateral loin pain occurred at 0100 hours (9 hours after the race), and he attended an emergency outpatient unit. Pentazocine hydrochloride was given by injection. Urinalysis showed no abnormalities, and the patient was negative for fecal occult blood. His serum amylase level was normal. On August 11, IVP suggested kidney hypofunction, but there was no stone in the urinary tract. A plain CT scan of the kidneys after 24 h showed bilateral patchy contrast enhancement (Fig. 7). A subsequent routine contrast-enhanced CT scan showed diffuse contrast enhancement immediately after the administration of the contrast medium, and bilateral wedge-shaped contrast enhancement 24 h later. The patient's urine volume was normal, and the loin pain persisted for 4 days.

A 24-year-old man (Patient 3). This patient had flu-like symptoms, and took a mixed preparation consisting of bucetin at 120 mg and aspirin at 240 mg. After 15 h, he participated in a 200-m race in an athletics meeting (October 10, 1980). After 6 h, he attended our hospital with nausea and bilateral loin pain. The severe pain, which made it impossible for him to drive a car, persisted for 2 days. His serum creatinine and urinary protein levels were 2.4 mg/dl and 2+, respectively, 4 days after onset. The patient was negative for urinary occult blood, and his urinary sodium level was 99 mEq/l. On the same day, drip infusion pyelography (DIP) revealed no ureteral

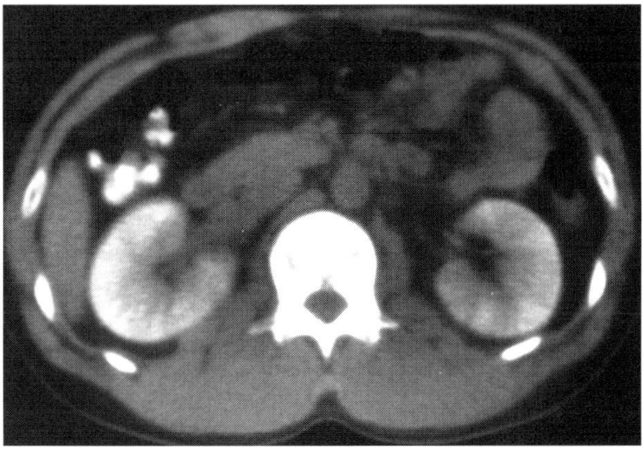

Fig. 6. Delayed CT 48 h after the administration of contrast medium. The serum creatinine level was high (5.5 mg/dl), and the contrast-enhanced areas were more extensive than those in Fig. 2 (serum creatinine 1.6 mg/dl). Patchy contrast enhancement changed to diffuse contrast enhancement

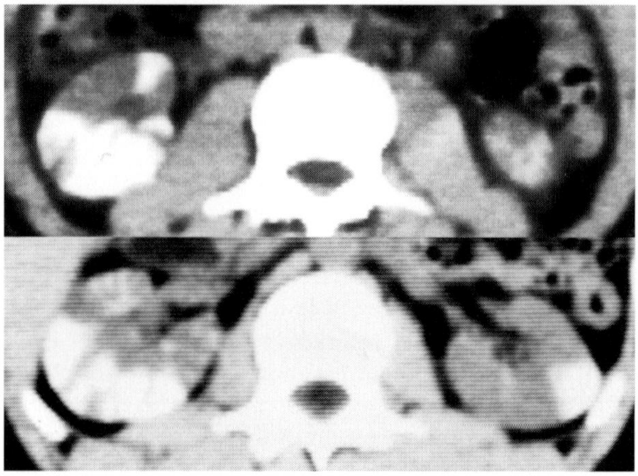

FIG. 7. Delayed CT 24 h after the administration of contrast medium (the *upper* and *lower* rows show different slices)

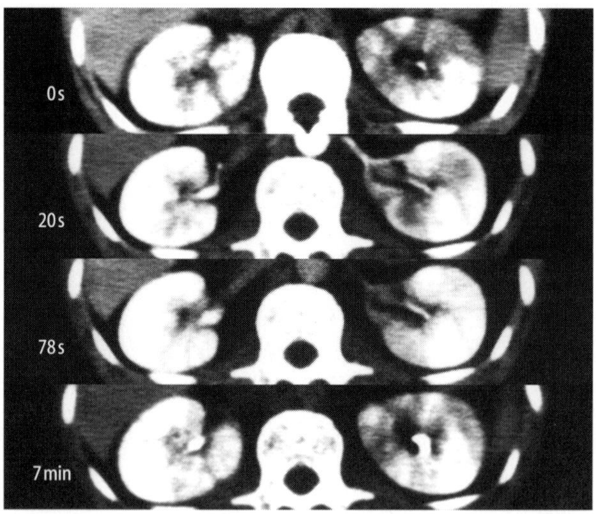

FIG. 8. Dynamic CT in the presence of wedge-shaped contrast enhancement (0 s)

stone, and kidney hypofunction was suggested. A CT of the kidney 6 h after the administration of a contrast medium showed patchy contrast enhancement in the kidney. In order to assess regional kidney function, dynamic CT was performed repeatedly within 3 min after bolus administration of the contrast medium (40 ml of 67% sodium iothalamate injected within 15 s through the anterior elbow vein) to investigate the process of contrast medium excretion [13]. The results are shown in Fig. 8 and in the analytical Fig. 14. Thirteen days after onset, the patient's serum creatinine level returned to 1.2 mg/dl.

A 35-year-old man, policeman. This patient took a single dose of aminopyrine at 375 mg, aminopropionic acid at 500 mg, and amoxicillin at 125 mg after pharyngeal pain had persisted for 5 days. After 2 h, nausea, vomiting, and loin pain occurred. On November 28, 1980, he attended an emergency outpatient unit at midnight with severe pain. Pentazocine hydrochloride was given by injection. On November 29, IVP was performed at 0300 hours after a tentative diagnosis of ureteral stone. However, there was no stone, and nephrograms were repeated. After 1 h, a CT scan of the kidney showed diffuse contrast enhancement (Fig. 9). However, plain CT after 21 h (delayed CT) showed patchy contrast enhancement, and this persisted for 45 h (Fig. 10). Furthermore, a CT scan of the kidney 1 and 1.5 h after oral administration

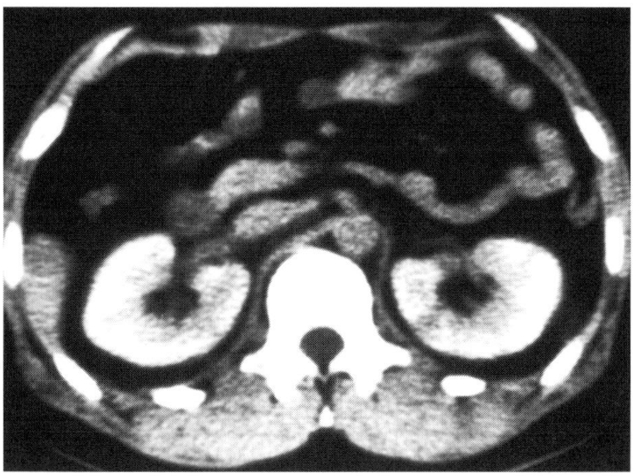

FIG. 9. Delayed CT 1 h after the administration of contrast medium (serum creatinine 3.3 mg/dl)

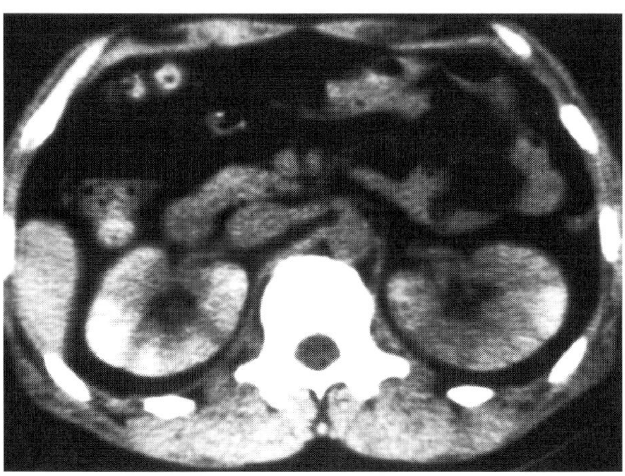

FIG. 10. Delayed CT 45 h after the administration of contrast medium

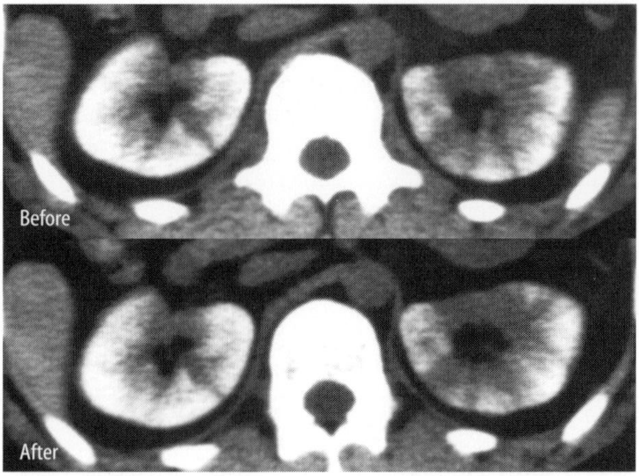

Fig. 11. Wedge-shaped lesions before and 1.5 h after the administration of SQ14225. There were no changes in the images (serum creatinine 3.6 mg/dl)

of an angiotensin-converting enzyme inhibitor (SQ 14225) at 125 mg did not reveal any changes (Fig. 11). The administration of SQ 14225 did not influence the patchy contrast enhancement, suggesting that SQ 14225 had not improved creatinine clearance. The patient's serum creatinine level was 2.8 mg/dl before IVP on November 28, and reached a maximum (3.6 mg/dl) 2 days after IVP, but gradually decreased to 2.1 mg/dl 4 days after IVP. Loin pain persisted for 5 days. His lactic acid dehydrogenase (LDH) level, serum myoglobin level, and urine volume were normal. Dark urine was not noted. His CPK level was slightly increased. Urinalysis showed that his urinary protein level was 1+, and was negative for occult blood.

In a text book on acute renal failure, published in 1982 [2], the four patients described above and the first ever patient were reported to have a new type of acute renal failure syndrome.

Chapter 3
Wedge-Shaped Patchy Renal Ischemia

1 Visualization of Residual Contrast Medium on Delayed CT in Relation to the Interval from the Administration of Contrast Medium (Assessment of Regional Kidney Function)

Contrast medium is filtered from glomeruli and excreted by the kidney. Owing to the differences in kidney function in local areas, a patchy lesion is visualized, not a diffuse lesion. We performed dynamic computed tomography (CT) in order to examine changes in the early phase after the administration of contrast medium (cortical phase, after 20–30 s). In areas with severe renal ischemia, contrast enhancement was less marked, and there was minimal cortical enhancement (the uptake of contrast medium was low at 3 min). However, in areas with mild renal ischemia, stronger contrast enhancement was observed. Delayed CT of a few hours and 1–2 days after the administration of contrast medium showed gradual wedge-shaped contrast enhancement in areas with severe renal ischemia (Fig. 12). However, in areas with mild renal ischemia, contrast medium had been excreted, and there was no contrast enhancement. The sites of contrast enhancement on CT were reversed a few hours and 1–2 days after the administration of contrast medium compared with those 3 min after administration [4] (Fig. 12). Wedge-shaped contrast enhancement was clearly observed on delayed CT 3 h and 1–2 days after the administration of contrast medium.

The mechanism by which wedge-shaped lesions were enhanced may involve renal vasoconstriction or tubular obstruction, as shown in Fig. 13. However, as bilateral multiple wedge-shaped lesions were detected, we considered that vasoconstriction was involved because vasoconstriction at the interlobar/arcuate artery level (Fig. 13-1) may be more probable than tubular obstruction in the papillary region (Fig. 13-2). Briefly, a serial increase in the level of contrast medium in severe lesions is similar to the delayed appearance time and hyperconcentration shown in a later film on the stenosed side of the kidney by rapid intravenous pyelography in a patient with renal artery stenosis. Contrast enhancement persisted for a few days, possibly because renal vasoconstriction extended the reduced glomerular filtration rate (GFR) in the area of severe renal ischemia. The small volume of contrast medium which filtered through

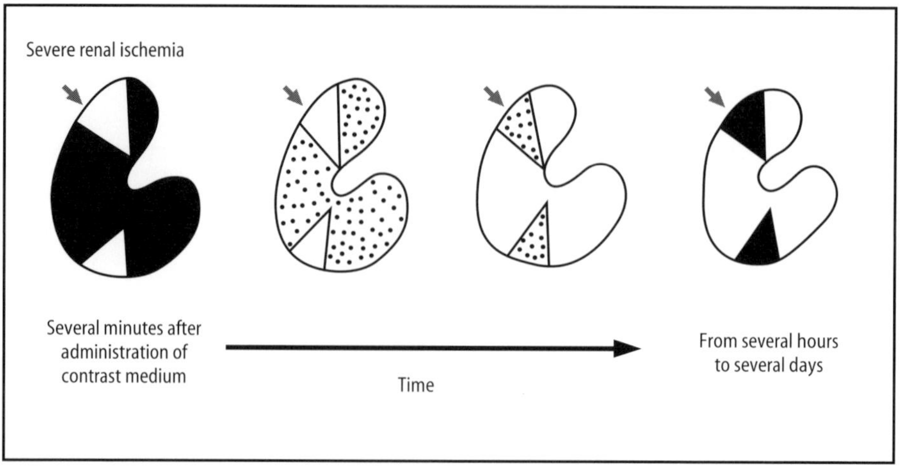

Fig. 12. Relationship between the interval after the administration of contrast medium and wedge-shaped contrast enhancement (From [4], with permission)

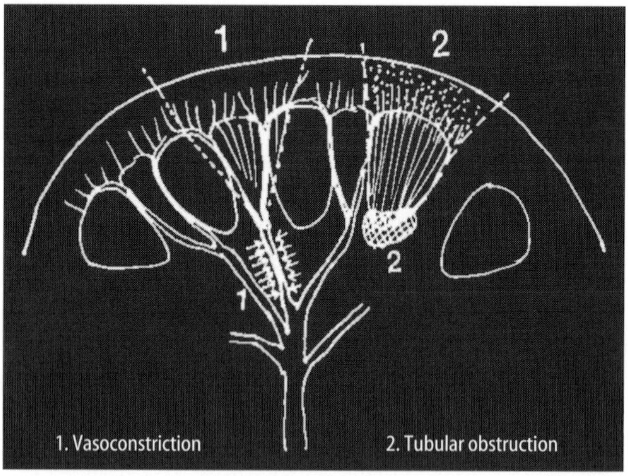

Fig. 13. Mechanism involved in wedge-shaped lesions

during this period may have been concentrated in the renal tubules, resulting in hyperconcentration. However, if tubular obstruction is involved in the mechanism, multiple lesions obstructing several collecting tubules simultaneously must develop in the bilateral kidneys. No study has reported patchy wedge-shaped contrast enhancement even in patients with tubular obstruction due to uric acid crystals (acute uric acid nephropathy).

2 Interpretation of Wedge-Shaped Renal Lesions

The area of wedge-shaped contrast enhancement increased with the increase in serum creatinine level. When the serum creatinine level exceeded 5 or 6 mg/dl, diffuse contrast enhancement involved the entire kidney. However, even in patients with diffuse contrast enhancement, delayed CT confirmed patchy wedge-shaped contrast enhancement again when the serum creatinine level decreased to 1.2–3.5 mg/dl in the recovery phase (refer to Patient 2 in Fig. 59, Chap. 10, Sect. 1). This finding in the recovery phase cannot be explained by tubular obstruction.

In order to compare kidney function between the areas where contrast persisted and those where contrast did not persist, we performed additional dynamic CT in a patient with wedge-shaped contrast enhancement [14] (Fig. 14, Patient 3).

We designed a method of evaluating regional kidney function [13]. First, 40 ml contrast medium was infused into the forearm vein within 15 s, and dynamic CT was performed at the same slice level at specific intervals. We confirmed the gradual transfer of contrast medium from the cortex to the medulla. We established the region of interest in the cortex/medulla, and serially investigated changes in the CT attenuation value in that region to evaluate kidney function (Figs. 15 and 16) [13]. The interval before the cortical curve crossed the medullary curve was correlated with glomerular filtration rate to some degree. In the area where contrast did not persist, the interval before the cortex curve crossed the medulla curve was nearly normal (Fig. 16), as shown in Fig. 14. However, in the area where contrast persisted on delayed CT, cortical/medullary contrast enhancement was less marked, and similar curves were noted. The kidney function was almost normal in the area where contrast did not persist, but was reduced in the area where contrast persisted [14]. In addition, the area where contrast did not persist on delayed CT showed no renal infarction.

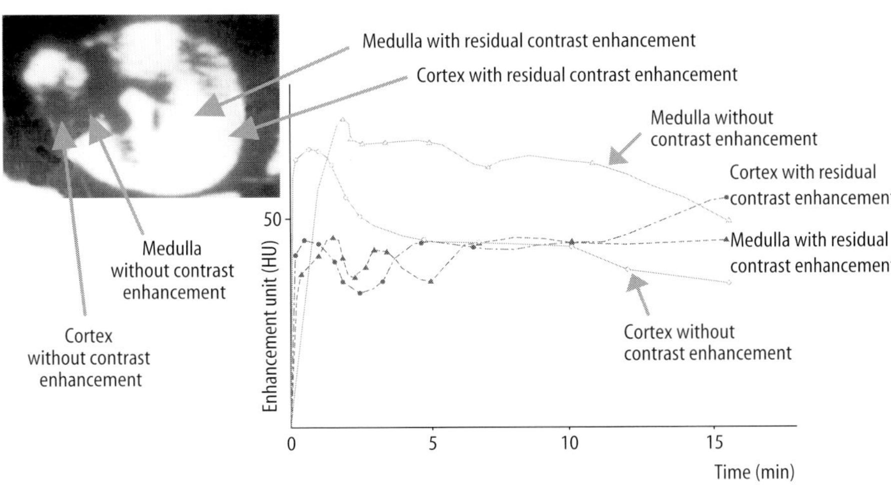

FIG. 14. Analysis of cortical and medullary curves by dynamic CT (comparison of function between the areas where contrast persisted and the areas where contrast did not persist) (From [14], with permission)

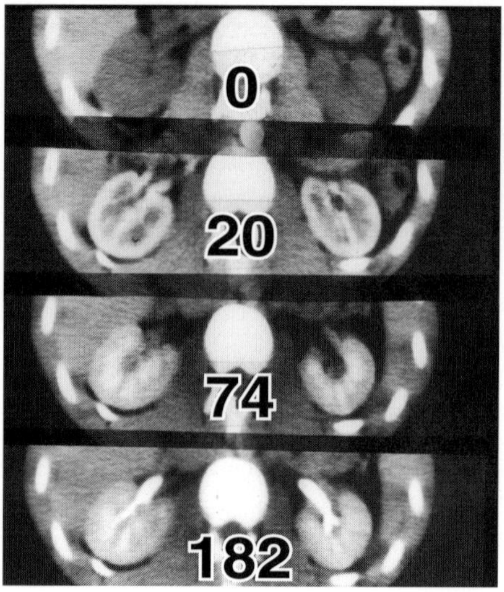

Fig. 15. Dynamic CT images in a person with normal kidney function (units: time (seconds) after the administration of contrast medium)

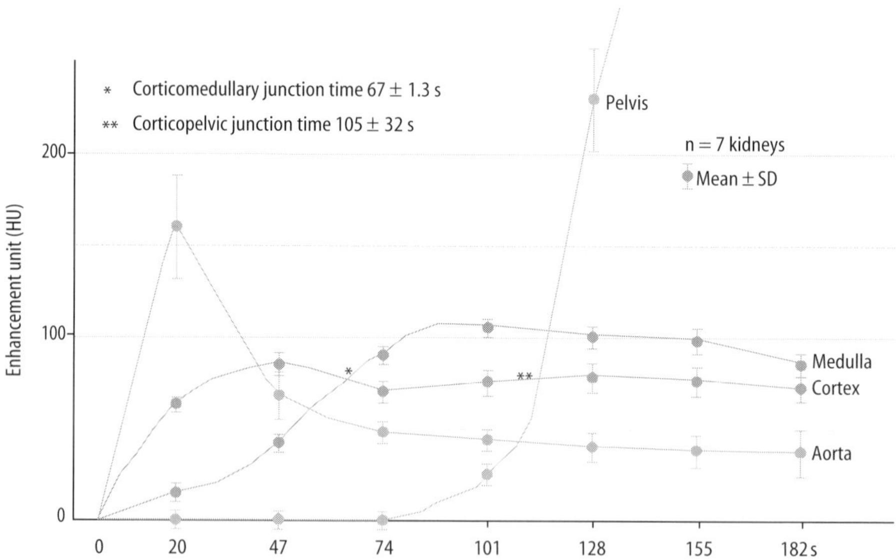

Fig. 16. Analysis of cortical and medullary curves by dynamic CT (people with normal kidney function) (From [13], with permission)

Subsequently, we examined whether it is only patients with exercise-induced acute renal failure (ALPE) who show wedge-shaped contrast enhancement [15–18]. We performed delayed CT on a patient with ALPE and a patient with myoglobinuric acute renal failure (due to a malignant syndrome) when their serum creatinine levels were 3.0 and 1.5 mg/dl, and compared the results. Wedge-shaped contrast enhancement was observed only in the patient with ALPE (Patient 19), and not in the patient with myoglobinuric acute renal failure. Diffuse contrast enhancement was noted (serum creatinine level, 3 mg/dl) (Fig. 17).

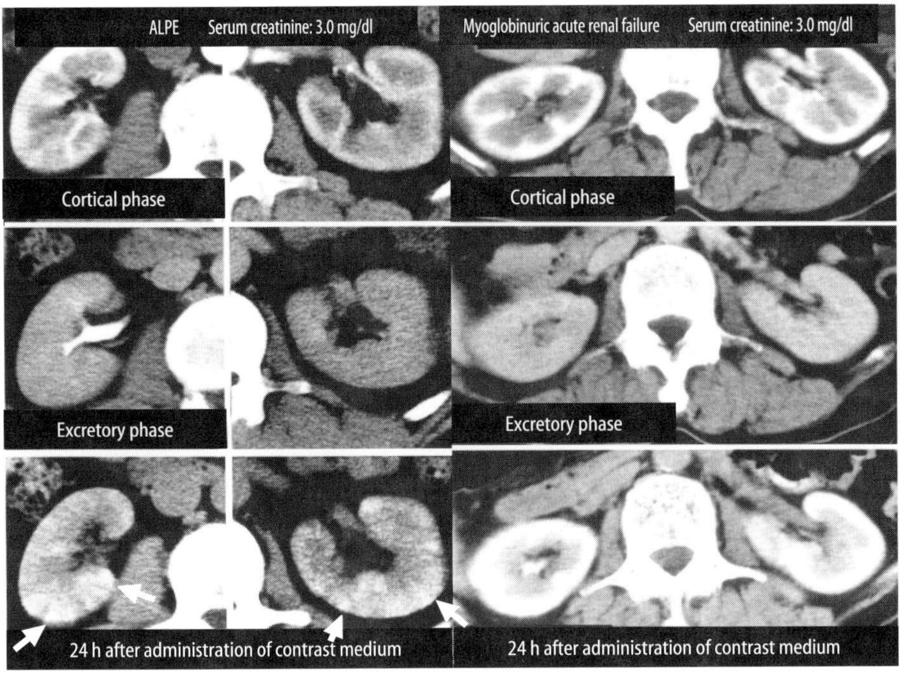

Fig. 17. Comparison of contrast enhancement 24 h after the administration of contrast medium between exercise-induced acute renal failure (ALPE) and myoglobinuric acute renal failure (serum creatinine 3 mg/dl). The patient with ALPE showed patchy wedge-shaped contrast enhancement, and the patient with myoglobinuric acute renal failure showed diffuse contrast enhancement

3 Administration of Contrast Medium in the Presence of Acute Renal Failure

After confirming the absence of dehydration, we carefully administered contrast medium at a reduced dose (40 ml) to patients with acute renal failure. We have not encountered any patient with an exacerbation of acute renal failure as a result of this treatment. Previous studies have indicated the safety of contrast medium in patients with acute renal failure, since it frequently induces overhydration, and thus differs from chronic renal failure [19,20]. However, another study reported that the administration of 100 ml contrast medium slightly prolonged the duration of oliguria [18]. When physicians hesitate to administer contrast medium in the presence of acute renal failure, a bone scan with ^{99m}Tc-methylene diphosphonate (MDP), magnetic resonance imaging (MRI) with gadolinium–diethylenetriaminopentoacetic acid (Gd–DTPA), and ultrasonography with Levovist can be performed. These procedures facilitate the detection of patchy lesions in some patients, although they are less sensitive than delayed CT.

4 Visualization of Wedge-Shaped Lesions by Bone Scan with MDP and MRI

Based on the finding that a bone scan with MDP showed muscular accumulation when rhabdomyolysis was marked [21], we performed this procedure on a patient. There was no muscular accumulation of MDP, but patchy accumulation was observed in the kidney, as shown in Fig. 18. This patient (Patient 5) was a physician in our department who had attended the Emergency Outpatient Unit for abdominal pain after skiing. His serum creatinine level was 2.0 mg/dl, and self-diagnosis suggested acute pancreatitis. However, 17 h after the administration of contrast medium, CT showed typical multiple wedge-shaped contrast-enhanced areas (Fig. 19). A bone scan with MDP accumulating in the ischemic site revealed a patchy accumulation of isotope in the renal ischemic site, which was consistent with the CT finding described above, and not in the muscle [22] (this photograph was printed on the cover of *Nephron*, see Fig. 20). However, in a bone scan with MDP, thick kidneys are visualized as 2-dimensional images, and this procedure is less sensitive in detecting patchy lesions than a CT scan. The course of this patient's condition is shown in Fig. 21. Some patchy lesions can be visualized by MRI in another patient (Fig. 22).

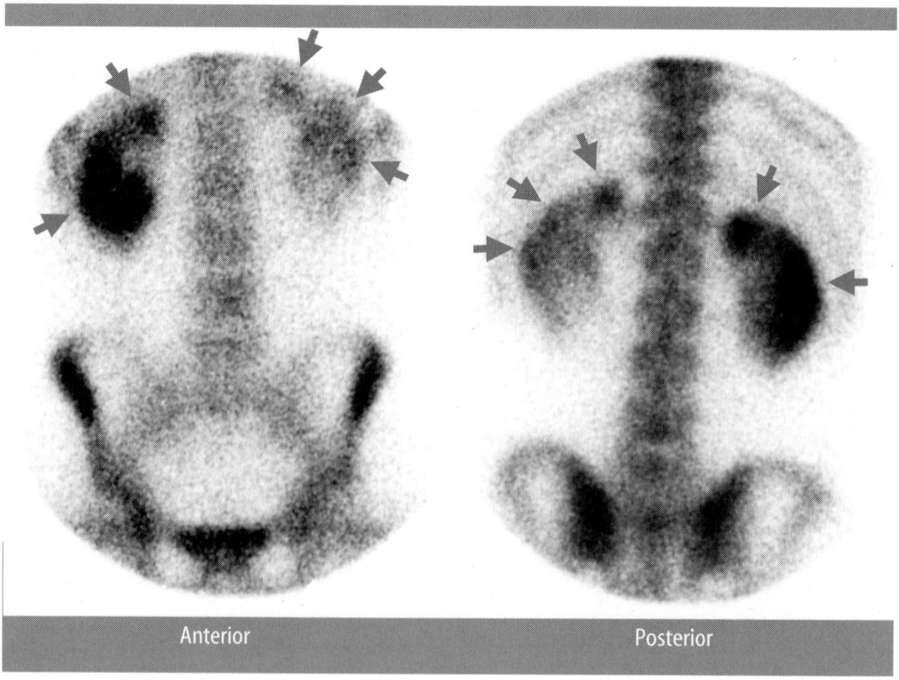

Fig. 18. Bone scan images with methylene diphosphonate (MDP). Patchy accumulation was observed in the kidney (From [22], with permission)

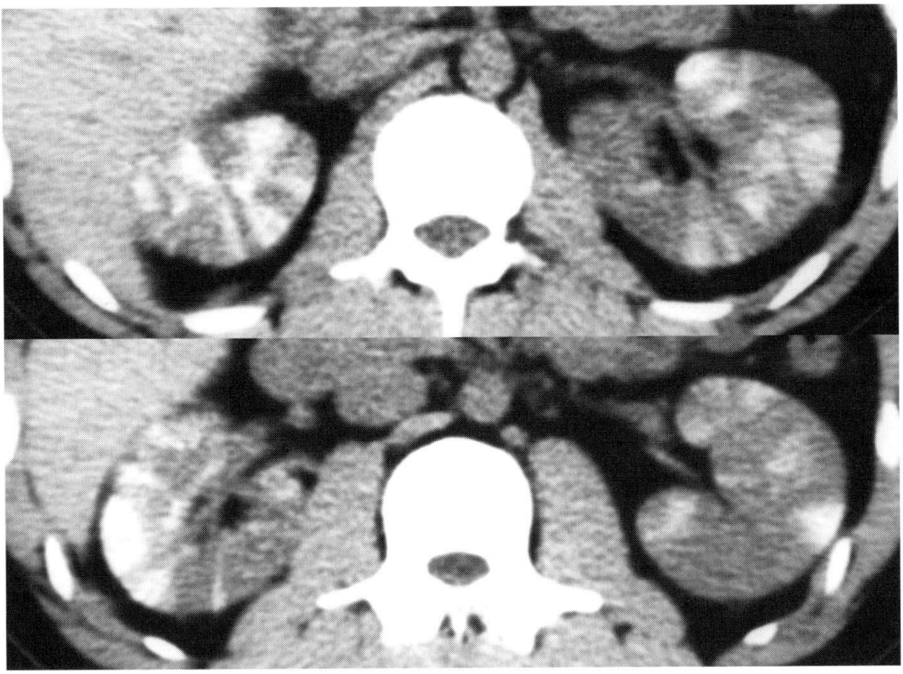

Fig. 19. Delayed CT 17 h after the administration of contrast medium to the patient in Fig. 18. Wedge-shaped contrast enhancement was observed in the bilateral kidneys (From [22], with permission)

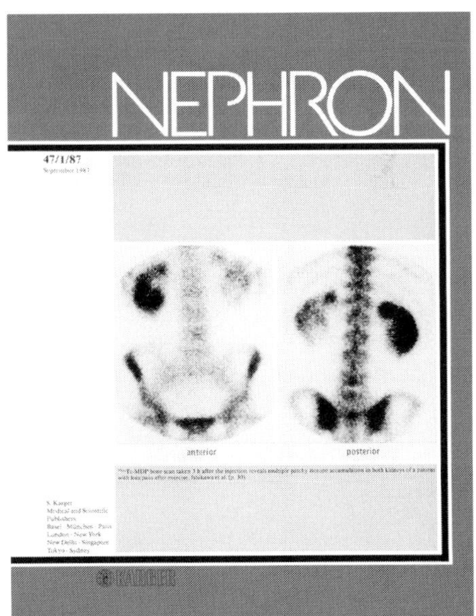

Fig. 20. MDP bone scan images in the patient in Fig. 18 were published on the cover of *Nephron* (From [22], with permission)

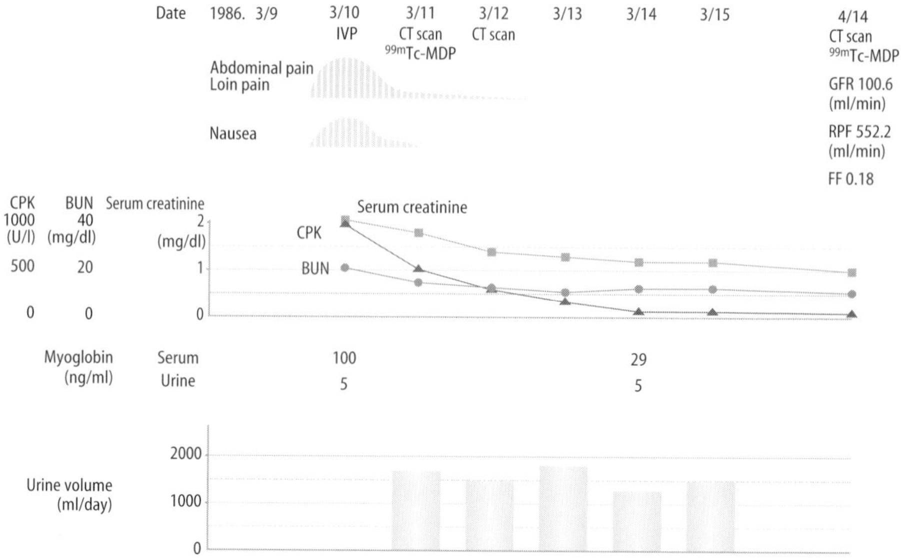

FIG. 21. Clinical course of Patient 5 (presented in Figs. 18 and 19)

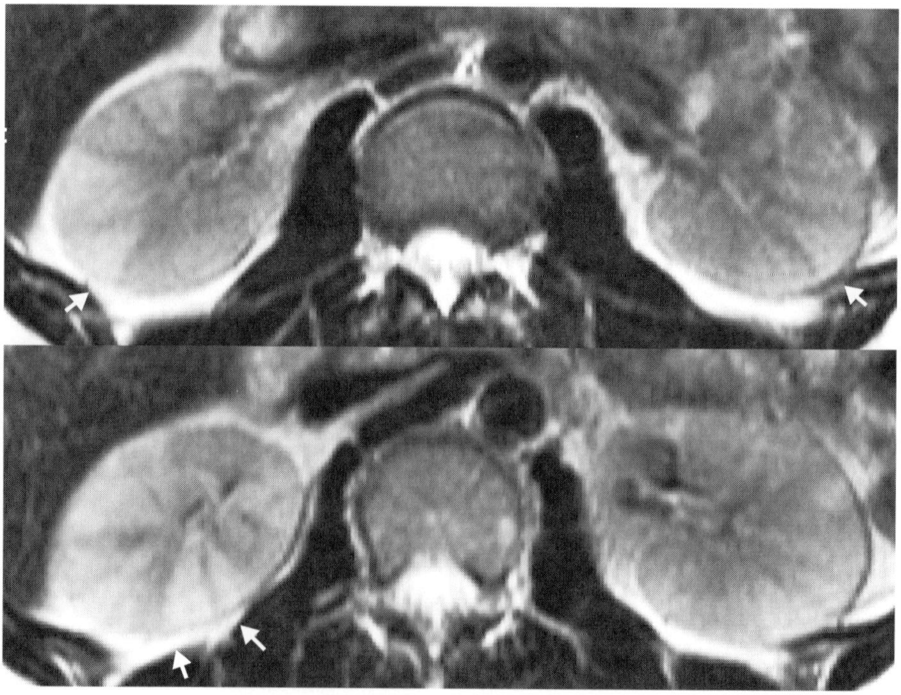

FIG. 22. Magnetic resonance imaging (MRI) without contrast medium showed wedge-shaped contrast enhancement in some patients (Patient 16; TR3600, TE138)

Chapter 4 Definition of Exercise-Induced Acute Renal Failure (ALPE)

1 Criteria for Typical ALPE

The criteria used in a diagnosis of ALPE are listed below.

1. Recent intense (anaerobic) exercise such as a short-distance sprint.
2. Mild rhabdomyolysis (which differs from that in myoglobinuric acute renal failure patients), and serum levels of creatine phosphokinase (CPK) and myoglobin, which are normal or slightly increased (less than 7 times the reference value for serum myoglobin, and less than 9 times the reference value for CPK).
3. Severe loin pain several hours after exercise.
4. Wedge-shaped contrast enhancement on plain CT from a few hours to 72h after the administration of a contrast medium (however, delayed CT after administration of the contrast medium is not essential to making a diagnosis).

The selection criteria for data collection are shown in Table 2.

Using these criteria, we reviewed the literature to investigate whether similar cases were described. One of the cases reported by Jackson in 1970 met the criteria [7]. This patient was an English soldier. Acute renal failure developed with vomiting and loin pain after a 200-m sprint and a 100-m race (Fig. 23). Severe bilateral loin pain persisted for 10 days. Jackson reported this patient as having myoglobinuric acute renal failure. However, he may have had ALPE. In Japan, in the case of a patient who developed muscular pain involving the right back to lumbar area and right lateral dorsal pain after a 100-m race, with a slight increase in CPK, Ueda et al. [23] reported that the patient had myoglobinuric acute renal failure. However, this patient may also have had ALPE.

In relation to the term "exercise-induced acute renal failure," this disorder was expressed as "loin pain and acute renal failure after exercise (athletics meeting)" in 1981 [24] (Fig. 24). Later, however, Nishimura and Takahara [25], Ishii et al. [26], and Nakamura et al. [27] named this disorder "exercise-induced acute renal failure." Since then, this term has commonly been used [3].

Table 2. Exercise-induced acute renal failure (ALPE)

Selection criteria	
(1) Intense (anaerobic) exercise such as a short-distance sprint	
(2) CPK less than 9 times and serum myoglobin less than 7 times the reference values	
(3) Acute renal failure with severe loin pain	
Patient with (1), (2), and (3)	
Total number of patients	155

CPK, creatine phosphokinase

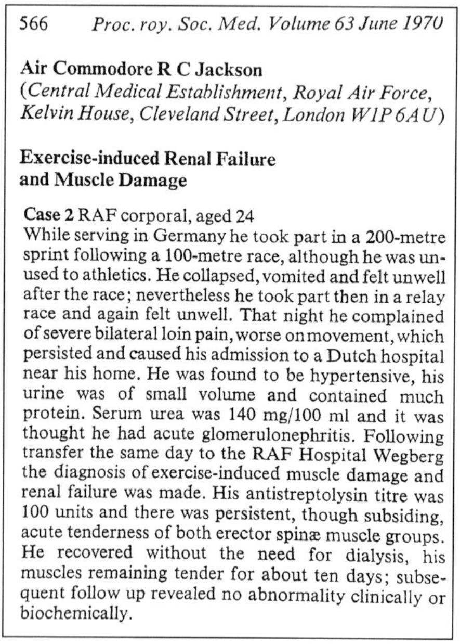

566 *Proc. roy. Soc. Med. Volume 63 June 1970*

Air Commodore R C Jackson
(*Central Medical Establishment, Royal Air Force, Kelvin House, Cleveland Street, London W1P 6AU*)

Exercise-induced Renal Failure and Muscle Damage

Case 2 RAF corporal, aged 24
While serving in Germany he took part in a 200-metre sprint following a 100-metre race, although he was unused to athletics. He collapsed, vomited and felt unwell after the race; nevertheless he took part then in a relay race and again felt unwell. That night he complained of severe bilateral loin pain, worse on movement, which persisted and caused his admission to a Dutch hospital near his home. He was found to be hypertensive, his urine was of small volume and contained much protein. Serum urea was 140 mg/100 ml and it was thought he had acute glomerulonephritis. Following transfer the same day to the RAF Hospital Wegberg the diagnosis of exercise-induced muscle damage and renal failure was made. His antistreptolysin titre was 100 units and there was persistent, though subsiding, acute tenderness of both erector spinæ muscle groups. He recovered without the need for dialysis, his muscles remaining tender for about ten days; subsequent follow up revealed no abnormality clinically or biochemically.

Fig. 23. A copy of the sentences suggesting ALPE in Jackson's study (From [7], with permission)

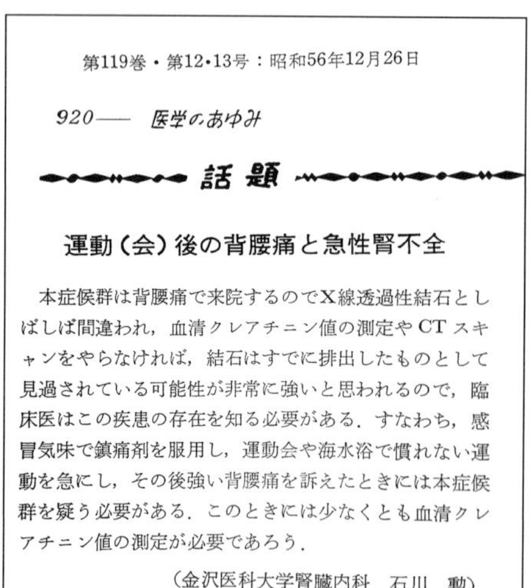

第119巻・第12・13号：昭和56年12月26日

920—— 医学のあゆみ

話 題

運動（会）後の背腰痛と急性腎不全

本症候群は背腰痛で来院するのでX線透過性結石としばしば間違われ，血清クレアチニン値の測定やCTスキャンをやらなければ，結石はすでに排出したものとして見過されている可能性が非常に強いと思われるので，臨床医はこの疾患の存在を知る必要がある．すなわち，感冒気味で鎮痛剤を服用し，運動会や海水浴で慣れない運動を急にし，その後強い背腰痛を訴えたときには本症候群を疑う必要がある．このときには少なくとも血清クレアチニン値の測定が必要であろう．

（金沢医科大学腎臓内科　石川　勲）

Fig. 24. A copy of the description of ALPE published in *Igaku-No-Ayumi (J Clin Exp Med)*. "Topics: loin pain and acute renal failure after exercise (athletics meeting). When patients with this new syndrome come to an emergency room complaining of loin pain, they are often misdiagnosed as having radiolucent urolithiasis. When a patient complains of severe loin pain after unaccustomed violent exercise at an athletics meeting or during summer bathing, in particular after taking a nonsteroidal anti-inflammatory drug (NSAID) for flu-like symptoms, this new syndrome should be suspected. In addition, the patient's serum creatinine level must be measured." (From [24], with permission)

2 Nontypical Cases

Some patients have nontypical ALPE. Some do not clearly remember having exercised [1,28,29], and others do not complain of loin pain [30,31]. In addition, others concurrently develop myoglobinuric acute renal failure and exercise-induced acute renal failure (ALPE), and show the characteristics of both disorders [32,33].

In the first patient and the fourth patient in our initial series (p. 7), the association of ALPE with anaerobic exercise had not yet been recognized, and their medical histories may have been insufficient, or the patients may not have reported intense exercise over a short duration. In acute renal failure patients with loin pain of unknown etiology, the presence or absence of anaerobic exercise should always be ascertained when taking their medical history. Erley et al. [28] did not comment on exercise in their study. However, when Sato et al. inquired about exercise in 1998 [34], Erley et al. reported that the patient had undertaken exercise.

In this study, these patients were regarded as nontypical cases, and were excluded from our series/data.

Chapter 5
Our Series (22 Patients)

1 Patient Characteristics

We have encountered a total of 22 patients with exercise-induced acute renal failure [4], and our clinical findings are summarized in Table 3. In most patients their creatine phosphokinase (CPK) and serum myoglobin levels were normal or slightly increased. In no patient were these levels higher than 10–20 times the reference values, which is different from patients with myoglobinuric acute renal failure. The type of exercise involved was anaerobic exercise requiring instant power over a short duration, such as short-distance running (sprinting), a swimming race, or weightlifting. In particular, 50% of the patients developed acute renal failure after running at full speed (sprinting) in an athletics meeting, and this disorder was considered to be post-athletics meeting or post-anaerobic exercise acute renal failure. In 4 of the 22 patients, renal hypouricemia was observed.

Patient 1: a 28-year-old man

This patient was the first case in our series in which acute renal failure developed after an athletics meeting. After he had participated in a 200-m race, loin pain occurred, leading to acute renal failure. Delayed computed tomography (CT) showed diffuse to patchy contrast enhancement. The details are given in Chap. 2, Sect. 2.

Patient 2: a 24-year-old man

Loin pain developed 9 h after a 200-m swimming race, leading to acute renal failure. CT 24 h after intravenous pyelography (IVP) showed patchy contrast enhancement. The details are given in Chap. 2, Sect. 2.

Patient 3: a 24-year-old man

This patient developed exercise-induced acute renal failure (ALPE) after participating in a 200-m race in an athletics meeting on a Health-Sports Day. When delayed CT showed patchy contrast enhancement, dynamic CT was performed in order to evaluate regional kidney function. The details are given in Chap. 2, Sect. 2.

Patient 4: a 27-year-old man

This patient's serum creatinine level was 3.7 mg/dl, which was higher than the value in the first patient. The area of residual contrast enhancement was also larger

TABLE 3. Clinical findings in our 22 patients with exercise-induced acute renal failure (ALPE)

Patient No.	Age (years) Sex	Prodrome (flu-like symptoms)	Analgesics*	Exercise	Loin pain	Duration of pain (days)
1	28 Male	+	+	Athletics meeting 200 m	+++	4
2	24 Male	–	–	Swimming	+++	4
3	24 Male	+	+	Athletics meeting 200 m	+++	2
4	27 Male	–	/	Athletics meeting 200 m × 3	+++	3
5	27 Male	+	+	Skiing (2 h)	+++	2
6	16 Male	–	+	Weightlifting	++	7
7	17 Male	–	–	Athletics meeting 400 m	+++	6
8	22 Male	+	+	Athletics meeting 100 m × 2	++	1
9	24 Male	–	–	Athletics meeting 200 m	+++	5
10	31 Male	+	–	Athletics meeting 100 m × 2	+++	3
11	33 Male	–	–	Athletics meeting 100 m × 2	+	1
12	34 Male	–	–	Flying a light plane	+++	3
13	21 Male	/	/	Near drowning	++	/
14	15 Male	/	/	Baseball	++	/
15	26 Male	–	–	Athletics meeting 100 m × 2	+++	4
16	19 Male	–	–	Time trial 100, 400, 1500 m	+++	4
17	19 Male	–	–	Physical training	+++	7
18	41 Male	–	–	Athletics meeting 150 m × 2	+++	14
19	39 Male	–	–	Near drowning	+++	10
20	27 Male	–	–	Baseball (6 h)	++	5
21	14 Male	–	–	Athletics meeting 400 m × 2	+	9
22	16 Male	–	–	Badminton	+	7

Nausea/vomiting	Slight fever	Initial serum creatinine (mg/dl)	Maximum serum creatinine (mg/dl)	Duration of ARF (days)	Renal CT findings
+	+	2.8	7.1	20	Diffuse, patchy
+	+	/	/	/	Patchy
+	+	2.4	2.4	13	Patchy
+	+	3.7	3.7	9	Patchy
+	−	2	2.1	5	Patchy
+	+	1.2	1.2	3	Partially patchy
++	+	7.3	8.1	18	Diffuse to patchy
+	+	3.9	3.9	12	?Patchy
+	−	1.9	2.1	6	Patchy
+	/	/	4.2	19	/
+++	/	/	5	10	/
−	+	2.1	3	6	Patchy
+	+	1.5	1.8	7	Patchy
+	+	3.7	5.1	19	Diffuse
+	+	1.6	1.6	10	Patchy
−	+	2.1	2.6	7	Patchy
+	/	3.5	3.5	10	Patchy
−	/	3	3	24	Patchy
+	+	7.3	10.4	30	Patchy
+	+	3.4	4.2	14	Patchy
+	+	1.5	12.2	24	Patchy
−	+	1.3	1.5	8	Patchy

TABLE 3. *Continued*

Patient No.	Duration of enhancement on CT (h)	Oliguria	UOsm/UNa	FENa (%)	Dark urine
1	72	–	300/42	2.2	–
2	/	–	/	/	–
3	/	–	381/99	2.1	–
4	72	–	306/44	0.6	–
5	21	–	276/46	0.8	–
6	24	–	289/49	0.5	–
7	41	±	308/26	1	–
8	/	±	/71	1.5	–
9	48	–	369/49	0.6	–
10	/	–	/	/	–
11	/	–	/	/	–
12	36	–	274/31	0.5	–
13	/	–	408/84	2.2	–
14	/	–	448/7	0.1	–
15	48	–	388/58	0.5	–
16	96	–	257/35	0.3	–
17	24	–	228/63	0.2	–
18	48	–	292/14	0.4	–
19	24	–	170/33	12	–
20	24	–	267/18	0.5	–
21	72	+	206/54	5	–
22	/	–	159/30	0.7	–

*, Taken before exercise
UOsm (mOsm/l), UNa (mEq/l)
CT, computed tomography; ARF, acute renal failure

Serum myoglobin (ng/ml)	CPK (U/l)	Myoglobinuria	Kidney biopsy	Hypouricemia
88	292	–	+	–
/	/	/	–	–
274	1650	–	–	–
90	42	–	–	–
100	998	–	–	–
35	1323	–	+	–
85	250	–	+	+
/	73	/	+	+
120	930	–	–	–
/	/	/	–	–
/	/	/	–	–
70	52	–	–	–
40	116	–	–	–
/	/	–	–	–
49	312	–	–	–
67	329	–	–	–
75	696	–	–	–
67	242	–	+	+
420	355	–	–	–
47	530	–	–	–
/	428	–	–	+
/	459	–	–	–

(Fig. 25). He had run three 200-m races in an athletics meeting. Several hours later, vomiting and loin pain occurred. The pain became severe, and he attended an emergency outpatient unit during the night. The findings did not suggest myoglobinuria. A plain CT scan 24h after the administration of a contrast medium revealed multiple wedge-shaped contrast-enhanced areas. At one area in the left kidney (Fig. 25, arrows), kidney function was almost normal, and the excretion of contrast medium to the renal medulla was observed by dynamic CT.

Patient 5: a 27-year-old man (a physician in our department)

This patient was the first case of ALPE in which a bone scan with ^{99m}Tc-methylene diphosphonate (MDP) showed patchy findings (see Fig. 18) (the details are given in Chap. 3, Sect. 4). Severe abdominal pain developed after skiing. He consulted our hospital under a self-diagnosis of acute pancreatitis.

Patient 6: a 16-year-old male high-school student

This patient was the first case in which magnetic resonance imaging (MRI) revealed a patchy lesion (Fig. 26). Lumbar pain occurred after a weightlifting session, and he took 75mg/day diclofenac sodium for 1 week. However, he did not stop weightlifting. On December 7, 1985, fever, nausea, and vomiting occurred. On December 9, he attended our hospital with severe loin pain. His serum creatinine level had increased from 0.8mg/dl (before onset) to 1.2mg/dl. CT 5h after IVP showed several wedge-shaped contrast-enhanced areas in the right kidney (Fig. 27). After 4 days, MRI

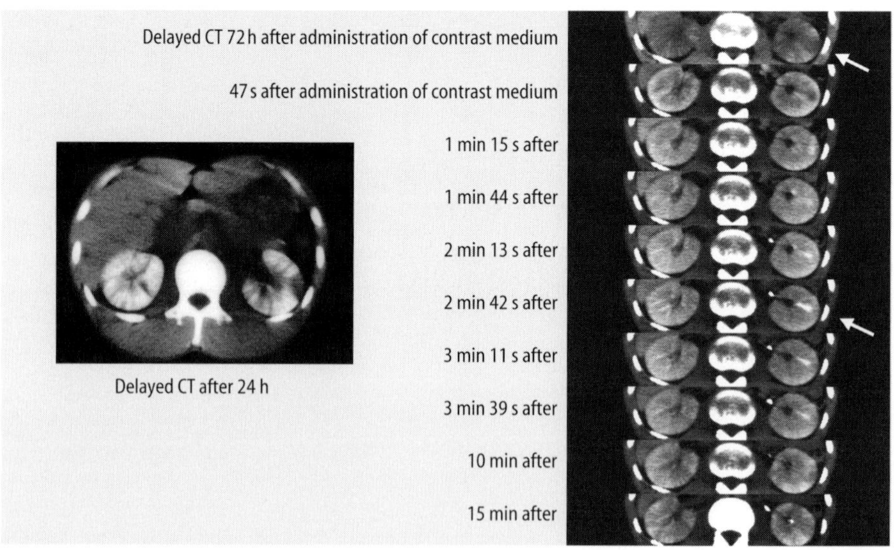

Fig. 25. *Left.* Delayed CT 24h after the administration of contrast medium. The area of contrast enhancement was more extensive than that seen at a serum creatinine level of 1.6mg/dl (Fig. 2) (From [41], with permission). *Right.* Dynamic CT in the presence of wedge-shaped lesions (72h after the administration of contrast medium). In a portion of the left kidney (*arrows*), the medulla was contrast-enhanced 2–3min later, suggesting that kidney function in this area was normal

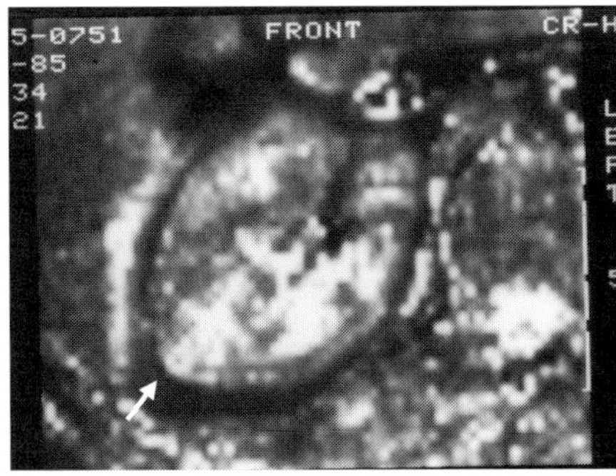

FIG. 26. A T1 time calculation image showing the prolongation of T1 at the lesion site (right kidney, *arrow*)

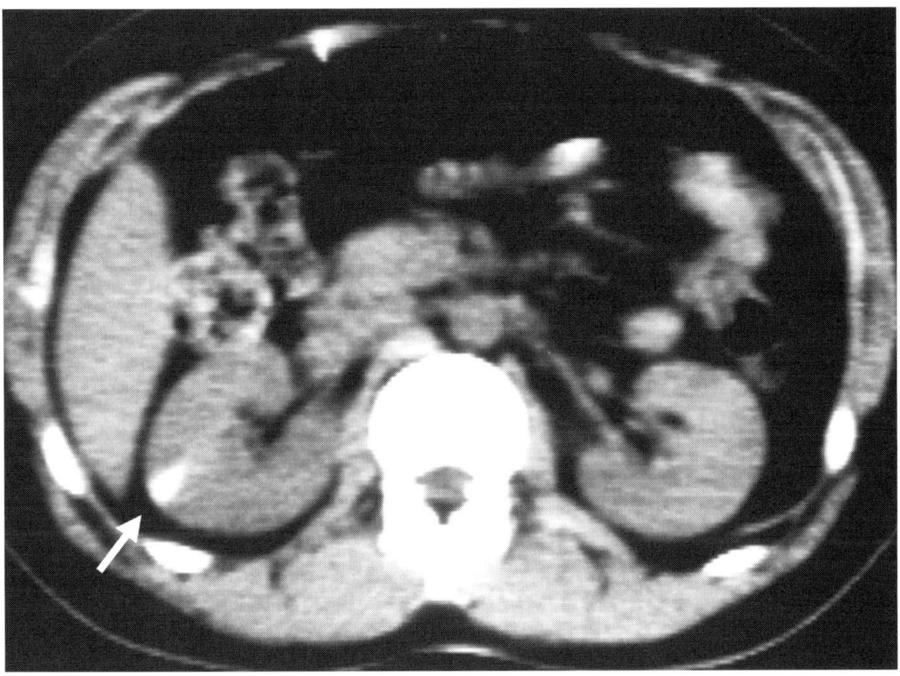

FIG. 27. Delayed CT. Wedge-shaped contrast enhancement was observed, which was consistent with the findings shown in Fig. 26

revealed low-signal-intensity areas that were consistent with the wedge-shaped contrast-enhanced areas on CT [35].

Patient 7: a 17-year-old male student

This patient was the first case in which ALPE developed in the presence of renal hypouricemia [3]. On September 26, 1984, he participated in a 400-m race in a school athletics meeting. On September 27, nausea and vomiting occurred about 12 h later at 0100 hours, and then bilateral loin pain and abdominal pain developed. Because

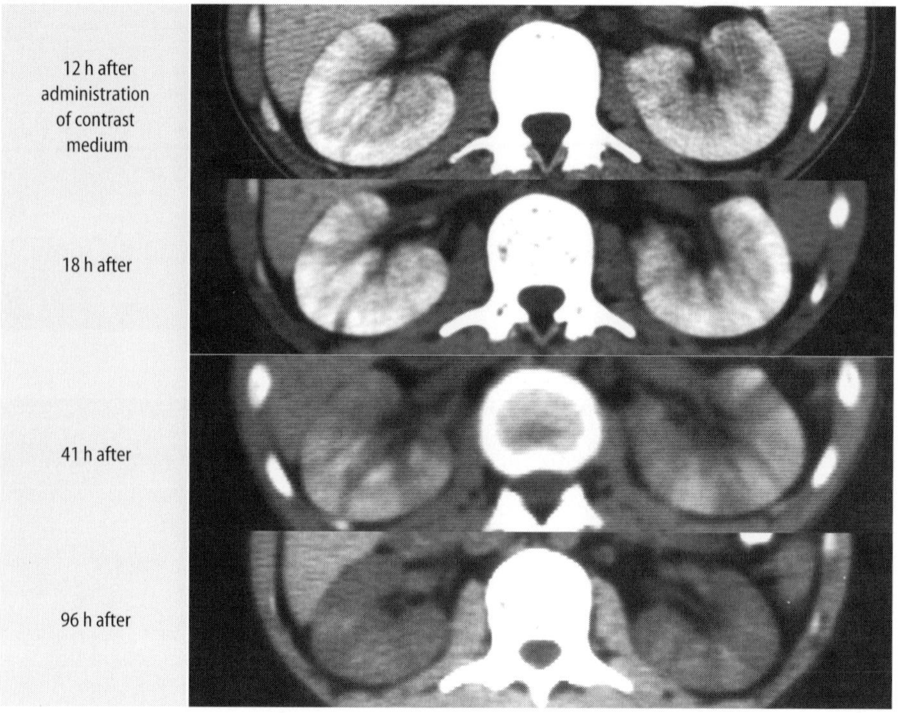

FIG. 28. Delayed CT 12, 18, 41, and 96 h after the administration of contrast medium. Patchy contrast enhancement persisted for 41 h

colicky pain persisted, he attended the Emergency Outpatient Unit of our hospital at 2200 hours on September 28. Bilateral knock pain at the costovertebral angle was marked. His urine color was normal, and his urinary protein level was 2+. Urinary sediment showed 40 erythrocytes per visual field. His serum creatinine and uric acid levels and fractional excretion of uric acid (FEUA) were 7.3 mg/dl, 5.5 mg/dl, and 28.7%, respectively. Delayed CT was performed 12, 18, 41, and 96 h after intravenous injection of 40 ml contrast medium (67% sodium iothalamate) on October 1. Diffuse to patchy contrast enhancement was observed in the kidneys (Fig. 28), which persisted for 41 h. The patient's serum creatinine level reached a peak of 8.1 mg/dl before the administration of contrast medium, but decreased to 6.7 mg/dl on October 2 after conservative therapy. His peak serum uric acid level was 5.6 mg/dl, but this decreased to 5.1 mg/dl on October 2. However, kidney hypofunction persisted for 18 days. On October 15, his serum creatinine and uric acid levels and FEUA were 0.9 mg/dl, 0.6 mg/dl, and 79.3%, respectively. A kidney biopsy on October 9 suggested that the acute tubular necrosis had healed. There was no uric acid deposition in the kidney tissue.

Patient 8: a 22-year-old man

This patient developed ALPE in the presence of renal hypouricemia [3]. He caught a cold, and took aspirin at 400 mg, ethenzamide at 150 mg, and acetaminophen at 300 mg on October 8 and 9, 1987. On October 10, he participated in two 100-m races at a district athletics meeting. After 4h, nausea and vomiting occurred. On October 11, malaise, loin pain, epigastric pain, and slight fever developed, and the patient attended a hospital on October 12. Urinalysis showed trace protein. However, his urinary sediment was normal, and his serum creatinine and uric acid levels were 3.9mg/dl and 2.7mg/dl, respectively. Thereafter, his serum creatinine level gradually decreased to 3.1mg/dl, 1.4mg/dl, and 1.0mg/dl on October 15, 19, and 27, respectively. However, his serum uric acid level also decreased to 1.7mg/dl, 1.0mg/dl, and 0.4mg/dl, respectively, suggesting renal hypouricemia. On October 30, the patient was admitted to our hospital for further examination. On October 17, 19, and 31, his FEUA values were 60%, 53%, and 58%, respectively (Fig. 29). On October 22, plain CT revealed swelling of the bilateral kidneys. However, the CT attenuation value in the medulla was not high, and there was no massive deposition of uric acid. Contrast-enhanced CT 10min after the administration of contrast medium showed no wedge-shaped contrast enhancement (Fig. 30). Thereafter, wedge-shaped contrast media enhancement was not attested. A kidney biopsy performed on November 4 revealed the healing stage of acute tubular necrosis. As the patient had renal hypouricemia, a test with benzbromarone and pyrazinamide was performed on November 12 to clarify the mechanism involved in the disordered kidney transport of uric acid. A presecretory reabsorption defect was suggested.

Patient 9: a 24-year-old man

This patient participated in a 200-m relay race at an athletics meeting on October 10. After dinner, a dull pain in his left flank occurred and gradually worsened, but it differed from colic. There was no decrease in urine volume or dark urine. At 2330 hours, the patient attended the Emergency Outpatient Unit of our hospital because of the pain. An intramuscular injection of scopolamine butylbromide relieved the

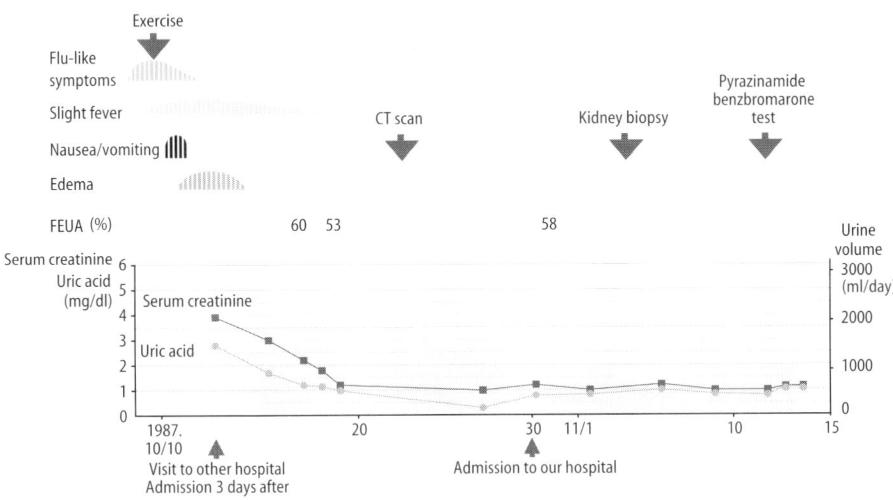

Fig. 29. The clinical course of ALPE complicated by renal hypouricemia

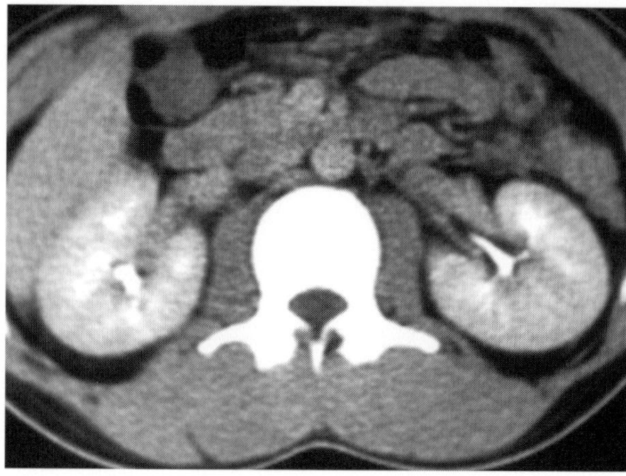

FIG. 30. CT 10 min after the administration of contrast medium. Wedge-shaped contrast enhancement was not clear

pain slightly. However, ureteral stone was suspected, and the patient was referred to our department. His serum creatinine and myoglobin levels were 2.1 mg/dl and 120 ng/ml (reference value, <60), respectively. Delayed CT after the administration of contrast medium on October 12 (Fig. 31) showed wedge-shaped contrast enhancement in the bilateral kidneys. On October 16 the pain disappeared, and on October 17 his serum creatinine level was 1.1 mg/dl.

Patient 10: a 31-year-old man

This patient developed loin pain after two 100-m races at an athletics meeting. In late May 1983, he caught a cold, but did not take any medication. On June 5, he participated in various events, including two 100-m races, at an athletics meeting. That evening, bilateral lumbar pain occurred, and he could not sleep. On June 6, the patient attended the Department of Orthopedics in our hospital. Under a diagnosis of lumbar pain, indomethacin suppositories were administered for 3 days. He attended the Department of Internal Medicine in our hospital on June 8. At the first visit, his blood pressure was 130/80 mmHg, and his body weight was 64.5 kg (3 kg weight gain). The patient was negative for C-reactive protein (CRP), plus/minus for urinary protein, and positive for occult blood. His serum creatinine and uric acid levels were 4.2 mg/dl and 14.7 mg/dl, respectively, but decreased to 1.4 mg/dl and 7.0 mg/dl, respectively, on June 17. On June 24, his serum creatinine level was 1.2 mg/dl. On June 30, his body weight returned to 61.5 kg.

Patient 11: a 33-year-old man

This patient was the first case in our series in which ALPE was detected with acute renal failure due to unknown etiology. On September 19, 1976, he ran two 100-m races at an athletics meeting. On September 20, vomiting, diarrhea, and upper abdominal pain developed, and the patient attended our department. His serum creatinine and uric acid levels were 5.0 mg/dl and 17.0 mg/dl, respectively. The pain persisted for 1

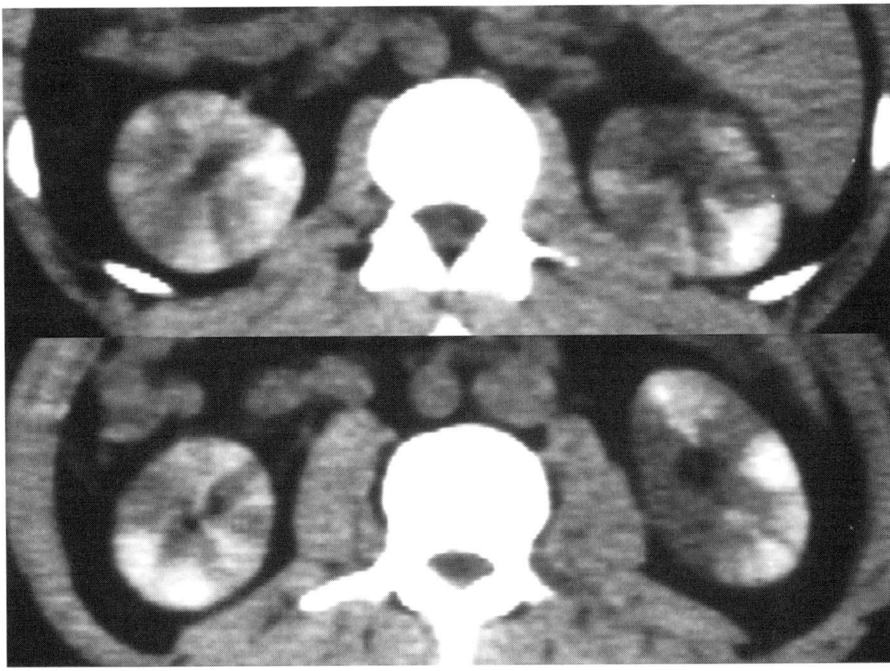

Fig. 31. Delayed CT 20 h after the administration of contrast medium. Wedge-shaped contrast enhancement was noted in the bilateral kidneys (the *upper* and *lower* rows show different slice levels)

day. However, these levels decreased to 3.2 mg/dl and 9.6 mg/dl, respectively, on September 24, and to 1.3 mg/dl and 6.7 mg/dl, respectively, on October 1. IVP on October 8 revealed no abnormalities, which suggested acute interstitial nephritis. However, no kidney biopsy was performed.

Patient 12: a 34-year-old man

This patient was admitted to hospital because of minimal change nephrotic syndrome. While in hospital he went out for exercise. In October 1987, minimal change nephrotic syndrome recurred, and steroid pulse therapy achieved complete remission. He was then admitted for maintenance therapy with prednisolone at 25 mg and mizoribine at 100 mg. During this time, he left our hospital and made a flight in a light plane (cycling-type exercise) for about 1 h on December 14. After 16 h, loin pain occurred, and his serum creatinine level was 3 mg/dl. On December 17, delayed CT 12 h after the administration of contrast medium revealed many wedge-shaped contrast-enhanced areas in the bilateral kidneys (Fig. 32). A bone scan with MDP showed an uneven abnormal accumulation of an isotope in the parenchyma of the bilateral kidneys (Fig. 33). On December 21, his serum creatinine level returned to 1.1 mg/dl, and on December 25, neither kidney CT nor delayed CT showed any abnormal findings.

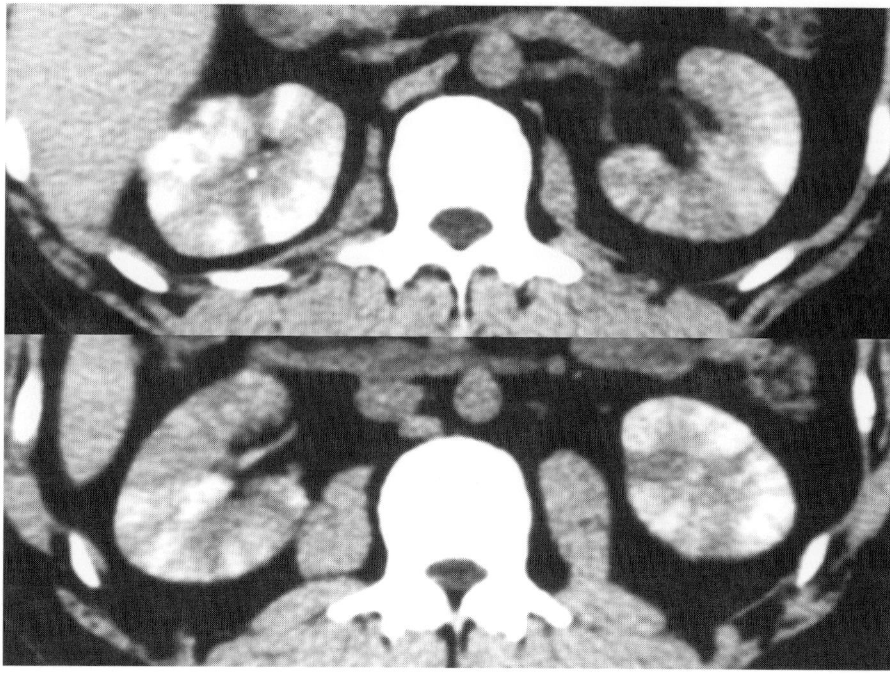

Fig. 32. Delayed CT 12h after the administration of contrast medium (the *upper* and *lower* rows show different slice levels)

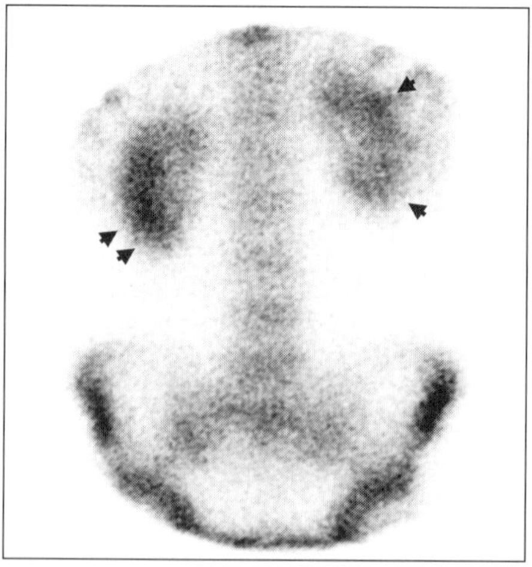

Fig. 33. Bone scan with MDP. An uneven abnormal accumulation of an isotope was seen in the parenchyma of the bilateral kidneys

Patient 13: a 21-year-old man

This patient, who had autosomal dominant polycystic kidney disease (ADPKD), almost drowned and then developed ALPE. On July 20, 1990, he nearly drowned in the sea at 1500 hours, and was brought to our hospital by ambulance for dyspnea and severe loin pain at 1620 hours. On admission, metabolic acidosis was observed. His CRP, serum creatinine, CPK, amylase, and urinary protein levels were 1+, 1.5 mg/dl, 116 U/l, 592 IU/l (derived from the salivary gland), and 2+, respectively. His body temperature was 37.7°C, and his blood pressure was 110/60 mmHg. His pulse and respiratory rate were 120/min and 22/min, respectively. Delayed CT 6 h after the administration of contrast medium showed wedge-shaped contrast enhancement in the noncystic renal parenchyma (Fig. 34). On July 24, a bone scan with MDP revealed patchy lesions (Fig. 35). His serum creatinine level was 1.3 mg/dl, which had decreased to 1.0 mg/dl on July 27. The patient was then discharged.

Patient 14: a 15-year-old boy

This patient was diagnosed as having acute enteritis. On May 31, 1993, upper abdominal pain occurred at the end of baseball training in the evening. After going home, severe pain, watery diarrhea, vomiting, and fever (until June 1) were noted. On June 1, he was diagnosed at a local clinic as having acute enteritis and underwent drip

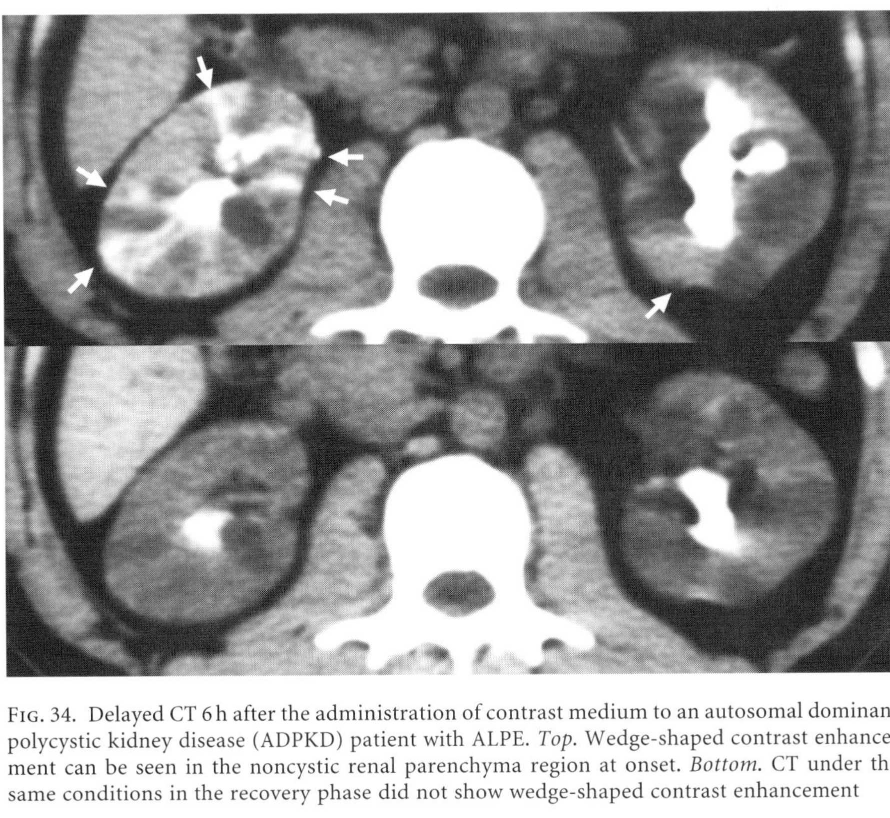

Fig. 34. Delayed CT 6 h after the administration of contrast medium to an autosomal dominant polycystic kidney disease (ADPKD) patient with ALPE. *Top*. Wedge-shaped contrast enhancement can be seen in the noncystic renal parenchyma region at onset. *Bottom*. CT under the same conditions in the recovery phase did not show wedge-shaped contrast enhancement

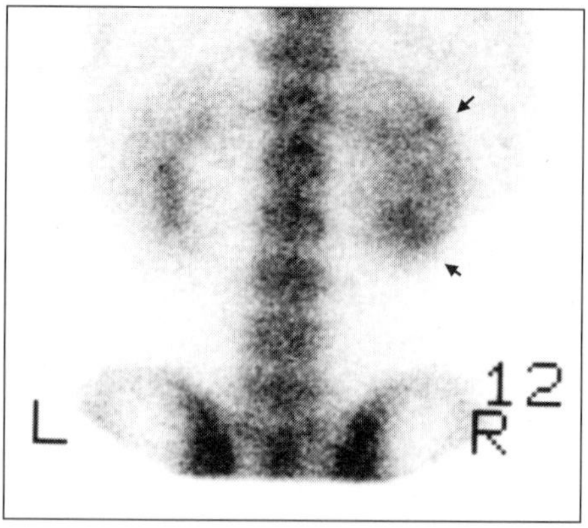

Fig. 35. Bone scan image with MDP in the same patient as in Fig. 34. A patchy lesion was observed. However, it was unclear whether this finding suggested ALPE or ADPKD

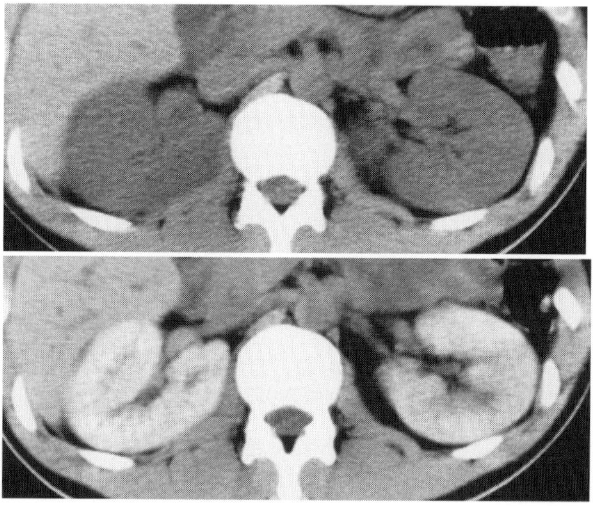

Fig. 36. *Top*. Plain CT showing a renal swelling (serum creatinine 3.7 mg/dl). *Bottom*. Delayed CT 18 h after the administration of contrast medium showed a diffuse uptake, although the patient's serum creatinine level had decreased to 1.8 mg/dl

infusion. However, on June 3, his serum creatinine level was 3.7 mg/dl. He was admitted to the local clinic, and treated with an antibiotic. On June 7, his serum creatinine level further increased to 5.1 mg/dl, and he was referred to our department. On admission, there were no changes in urine volume. His blood pressure was 140/60 mmHg, and his body temperature was 36.7°C. His serum creatinine, uric acid, UOsm, UNa, and FENa values were 4.3 mg/dl, 11.0 mg/dl, 448 mOsm/l, 7.0 mEq/l, and 0.1 %, respectively. On June 10 (recovery phase), delayed CT 18 h after the administration of contrast medium (serum creatinine level 1.8 mg/dl) showed diffuse contrast enhancement (Fig. 36). In our series, only this patient showed diffuse contrast enhancement with a serum creatinine level of 1.8 mg/dl. The reason why there was no patchy contrast enhancement was unclear. On June 22, his serum creatinine level decreased to 0.9 mg/dl.

Patient 15: a 26-year-old man

This patient, who had ADPKD, developed ALPE after a sprint. On October 1, 1995, he participated in two 100-m races at an athletics meeting in the morning. After a few hours, severe loin pain occurred, and he attended our department the following morning. There were no other abnormal findings, and his blood pressure, pulse, and serum creatinine values were 120/66 mmHg, 64/min, and 1.6 mg/dl (serum creatinine level before onset 0.9 mg/dl), respectively. On October 2, delayed CT 4 and 24 h after the administration of contrast medium showed patchy lesions (Fig. 37). On October 14, his serum creatinine level returned to 1.1 mg/dl, and CT 4 h after the administration of contrast medium showed no contrast enhancement.

Patient 16: a 19-year-old man

On June 13, 1998, this patient participated in 100-m, 400-m, and 1500-m time-trial races at 1400 hours. Left loin pain occurred at 1600 hours. He considered that he had caught a cold, and took a commercially available drug for colds and an analgesic agent. Initially, pain was marked in the sitting position, and became less marked in the supine position. However, it gradually became worse even in the supine position, and he attended the Emergency Outpatient Unit of our hospital at 0500 hours on June 14. His serum creatinine, total bilirubin, and CPK levels were increased to 2.1 mg/dl, 2.8 mg/dl (the reason for an increase in total bilirubin was unclear), and 329 U/L, respectively, and the patient was referred to our department. On June 14, CT 24, 48, and 96 h after the administration of contrast medium showed patchy lesions (Fig. 38)

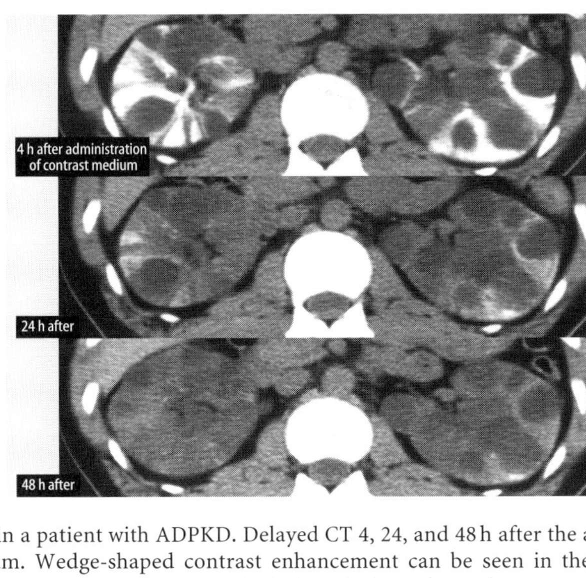

Fig. 37. ALPE in a patient with ADPKD. Delayed CT 4, 24, and 48 h after the administration of contrast medium. Wedge-shaped contrast enhancement can be seen in the noncystic renal parenchyma. This finding was more marked after 4 h than after 24 h

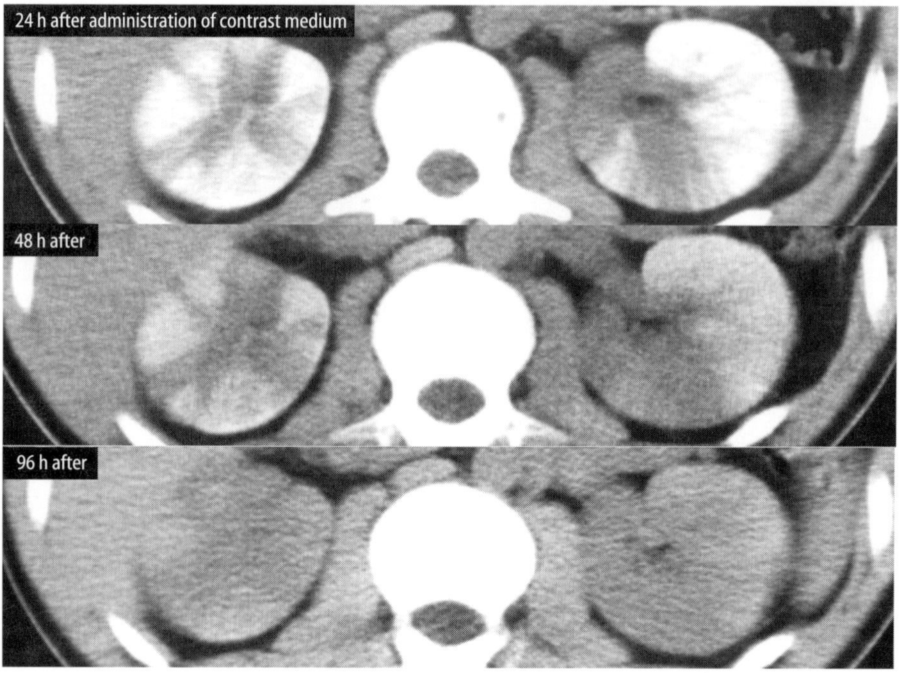

Fig. 38. Delayed CT 24, 48, and 96 h after the administration of contrast medium

(serum creatinine level 2.6 mg/dl). On June 17, T2-weighted images (T2WI) on MRI revealed patchy changes in signal intensity without contrast medium (see Fig. 22). Patchy lesions could be visualized by dynamic MRI (Fig. 39) and by a bone scan with MDP (Fig. 40).

Patient 17: a 19-year-old man

This patient was treated under a diagnosis of acute enteritis. He participated in festival training, such as running and jumping with sticks, for 4 h per day from August 16 until August 20, 1998. On August 18, abdominal pain occurred, followed by nausea on August 19. He attended a local clinic, and was treated under a diagnosis of acute enteritis. However, on August 20, the abdominal pain became worse, and he attended the Emergency Outpatient Unit of our hospital at 2200 hours. His serum creatinine level had increased to 3.5 mg/dl. On August 22, delayed CT showed patchy lesions (Fig. 41). On August 25, his serum creatinine level returned to 1.2 mg/dl.

Patient 18: a 41-year-old man

This patient (Case 1 in Fig. 57) and his son developed ALPE in the presence of renal hypouricemia [36]. After two 150-m sprints and rope skipping (40 skips) in a town athletics meeting, he developed ALPE. Gene analysis was performed to check for renal hypouricemia. The patient's son also developed ALPE (Case 2 in Fig. 57). The details are given in Chap. 10, Sect. 1.

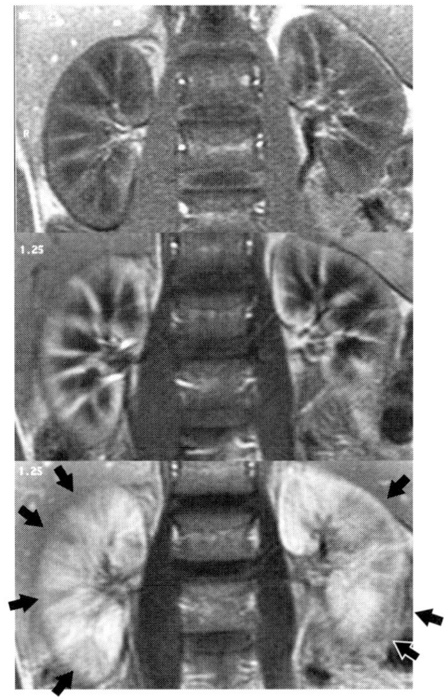

FIG. 39. MRI before and after the administration of Gd–DTPA. *Upper row*, before the administration of Gd–DTPA (TR 11.0, TE 4.2/1). *Middle row*, 2 min after the bolus administration of Gd–DTPA at 15 ml (TR 110, TE 4.1/1). *Lower row*, 4 min after the bolus administration (TR 110, TE 4.1/1). At the *arrows* in the *lower row*, the uptake of Gd–DTPA was low in some areas

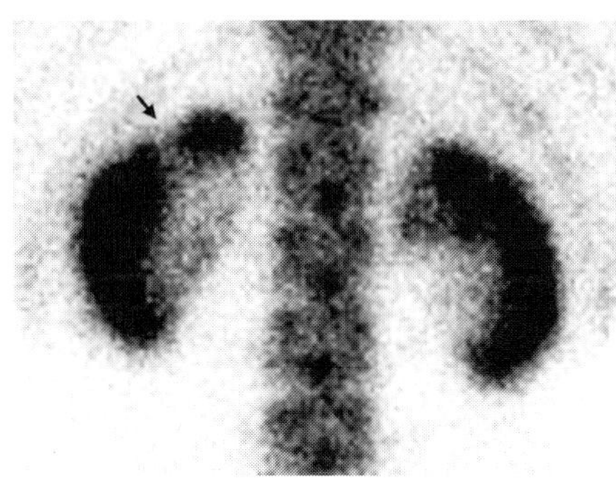

FIG. 40. Bone scan with MDP. The patchy findings were more marked in the left kidney

Patient 19: a 39-year-old man

This patient required hemodialysis for ALPE. Delayed CT and a bone scan with MDP in the recovery phase showed patchy lesions (these imaging procedures were performed in conjunction with another patient with myoglobinuric acute renal failure due to a malignant syndrome). On July 19, 1999, the patient fell into the water while fishing in a mountain stream, and was carried about 100 m in a few minutes while struggling all the time. As a precaution, he was admitted to a local clinic overnight. There were no abnormal laboratory data. However, at 0300 hours on July 21, he attended the Emergency Outpatient Unit of our hospital with severe bilateral loin

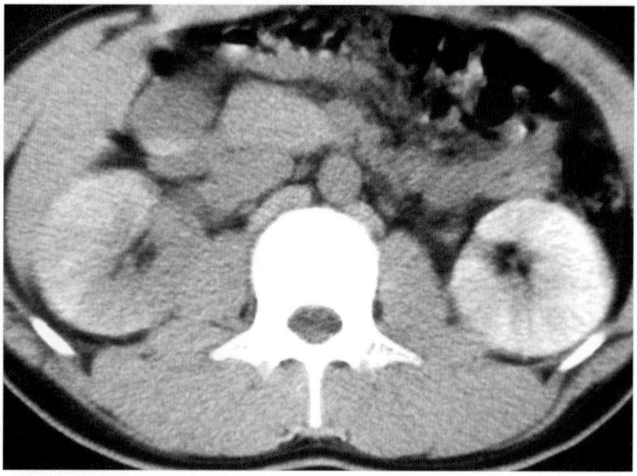

Fig. 41. Delayed CT 21 h after the administration of contrast medium. Patchy contrast enhancement can be seen

pain. His serum creatinine level was 7.3 mg/dl. Under a diagnosis of ALPE, he was admitted to our hospital and hemodialysis was performed. On August 16, his serum creatinine level returned to 1.2 mg/dl. CT on July 31 revealed patchy lesions (Fig. 42).

Patient 20: a 27-year-old man

In this case, ALPE was complicated by nocturnal hemoglobinuria. At the age of 20 years, the patient developed nocturnal hemoglobinuria. He had been treated in the Department of Hematology and Immunology in our hospital. On June 18, 2000, he participated in a practice baseball game from 0900 hours until 1500. At 1700 hours, right abdominal and loin pain occurred. On June 19, his serum creatinine level was 3.4 mg/dl (before onset, 0.7 mg/dl). On June 22, CT 24 h after the administration of contrast medium showed patchy lesions (Fig. 43). On June 26, his serum creatinine level had returned to 1.2 mg/dl.

Patient 21: a 14-year-old boy

This patient and his father (Patient 18) developed ALPE in the presence of renal hypouricemia [36] (Case 2 in Fig. 57). The son developed ALPE after participating in two 400-m races, a mock cavalry battle, and a tug of war in an athletics meeting. At a local clinic, a nonsteroidal anti-inflammatory drug (NSAID) was administered orally under a diagnosis of "muscular pain," and the condition was exacerbated. Gene

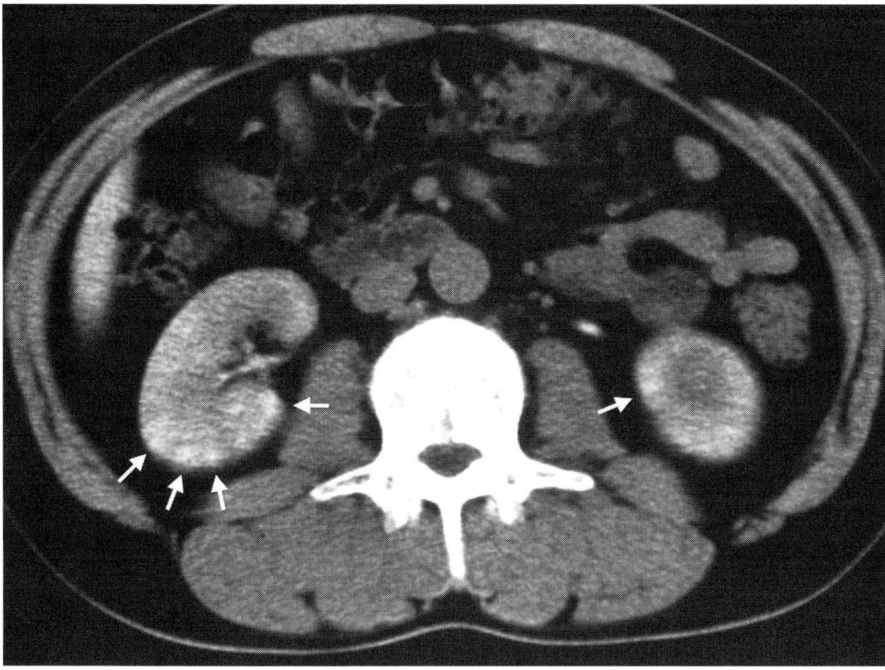

FIG. 42. Delayed CT 24 h after the administration of contrast medium. Patchy contrast enhancement can be seen in the right kidney

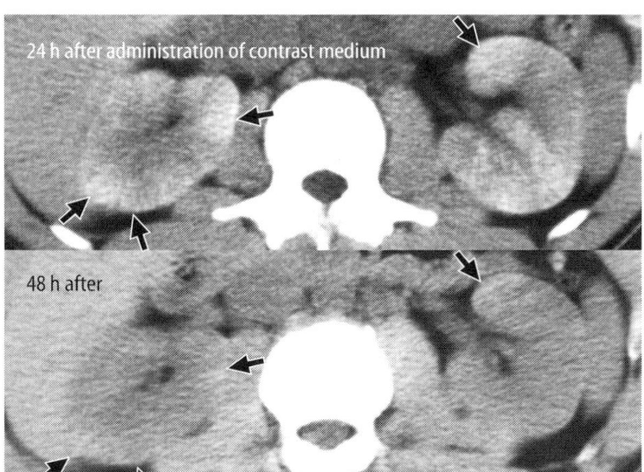

FIG. 43. Delayed CT 24 and 48 h after the administration of contrast medium. Contrast enhancement can be detected 48 h after administration, although it is less marked

analysis was performed, and MRI revealed patchy lesions. The details are given in Chap. 10, Sect. 1.

Patient 22: a 16-year-old male high-school student

In this patient, acute pyelonephritis was suspected in the presence of mycoplasma pneumonia. At the age of 12 years, he developed fever and loin pain, and was treated under a diagnosis of acute right pyelonephritis. After entering high school, he joined the badminton team. He trained for 4 h or more per day from January 4, 2005. On January 8, he felt very hot during training, and took an antipyretic analgesic for fever (40°C) after exercise. He then stayed at home. However, on January 10, loin pain occurred. The pain did not subside, and he attended a local clinic. Under a tentative diagnosis of acute pyelonephritis, the patient was referred to our department on January 11. On admission, his CRP level was increased to 6.1 mg/dl. He was positive for urinary protein and occult blood. There were no leukocytes in the urinary sediment. Furthermore, his serum creatinine level was 1.3 mg/dl, suggesting kidney dysfunction. His CPK level was slightly increased at 459 U/l. The administration of a cephem antibiotic did not relieve the fever. CT 4 h after the administration of contrast medium showed multiple wedge-shaped contrast-enhanced areas in the bilateral kidneys (Fig. 44). In addition, an infiltrating shadow in the left inferior lung field suggested mycoplasma pneumonia, and the agent was switched to a macrolide antibiotic, after which the pneumonia rapidly subsided. His serum creatinine level reached a maximum (1.5 mg/dl) 4 days after admission, but then decreased to 0.9 mg/dl at discharge. After the patient's condition had improved, CT showed no wedge-shaped contrast enhancement in the kidneys. The mycoplasma pneumonia may have caused the fever, which was complicated by ALPE.

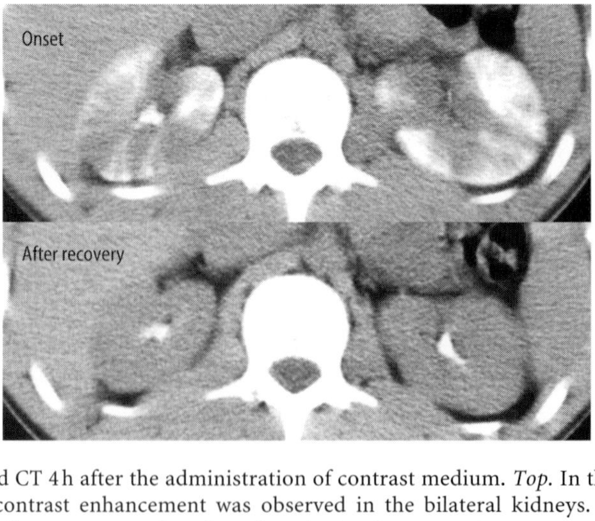

Fig. 44. Delayed CT 4 h after the administration of contrast medium. *Top.* In the initial phase, wedge-shaped contrast enhancement was observed in the bilateral kidneys. *Bottom.* In the recovery phase, there was no wedge-shaped contrast enhancement

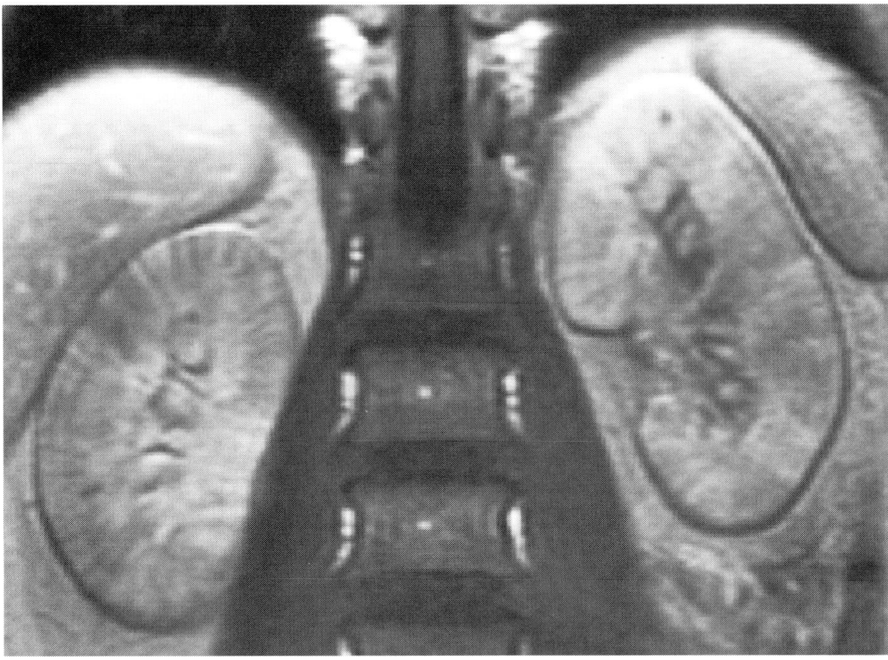

FIG. 45. MRI 3 min after the bolus administration of Gd–DTPA at 15 ml (TR 130.0, TE 4.1/1). Striated Gd–DTPA accumulation and low uptake can be seen in some areas

2 Delayed CT, MRI, and Bone Scan with MDP

In our series, we reviewed examples of wedge-shaped contrast enhancement. Many patients showed swelling of the kidney. Delayed CT showed wedge-shaped contrast enhancement from 3 to 24 h after the administration of a contrast medium, during which time the patient's serum creatinine level ranged from 1.2 to 3.5 mg/dl. After the patient's condition had improved, no swelling of the kidney or wedge-shaped contrast enhancement was observed in any patient under the same conditions, suggesting that the lesions were reversible.

MRI and a bone scan with MDP showed wedge-shaped contrast enhancement in some patients, although these procedures were less sensitive than CT. Patchy lesions could be visualized by a bone scan with MDP in Patients 5 (Fig. 18), 12 (Fig. 33), 13 (Fig. 35), and 16 (Fig. 40). This visualization was achieved by MRI in Patients 6 [35] (Fig. 26), 16 (Fig. 22 and Fig. 39), and 21 (Fig. 45). In the future, ultrasonography with Levovist will facilitate the visualization of lesions.

3 Kidney Biopsy

In 5 of the 22 patients, a kidney biopsy was performed. The findings suggested that these patients were in the recovery phase of acute tubular necrosis.

Chapter 6
Summary of 155 Cases Collected from the Literature

For this collection of data, we selected patients with acute kidney dysfunction or acute renal failure who met the above criteria for exercise-induced acute renal failure (ALPE), and who also matched our description. We collected a total of 155 patients with ALPE. The first 118 patients [2,3,22,27,30,34,35,37–95, Yamagata (personal communication, 1986), Ishikawa (unpublished results, 1994), Kadowaki (personal communication, 1996)] included 20 who we encountered before December 2000, and the remaining 37 patients [36,96–126] included 2 who we encountered between January 2001 and December 2004.

A summary of these 155 patients is shown in Table 4. We collected a total of 173 patients by adding 18 more patients [127–136] including 1 who we encountered before December 2005.

1 Background

The ages of the 150 patients whose ages were known ranged from 10 to 54 years, with a mean of 21.7 ± 7.8 years (Fig. 46). ALPE was particularly frequent in patients aged 14–25 years. Among 154 of the patients, 143 (92.9%) were male. It seems that males sprint more frequently than females.

Furthermore, 28 (46%) of the 61 patients in whom the presence or absence of a cold was recorded had caught a cold prior to exercise, and 23 (34%) of 68 patients took cold medicine or antipyretic analgesics (Fig. 47).

2 Findings and Laboratory Data on the First Visit

The findings for the patients on their first visit to a clinician included loin pain, nausea/vomiting (96%), and slight fever (76%) (Fig. 48). Among our patients, 18 (85.7%) of 21 patients were positive for C-reactive protein (CRP), 8 (38.1%) of 21 patients had hypertension, and weight gain was noted in 13 (65.0%) of 20 patients, suggesting overhydration.

The mean serum creatinine level on the first visit was 4.7 ± 2.8 mg/dl. The mean maximum serum creatinine level was 6.0 ± 3.1 mg/dl (Fig. 49, Table 4). The prognosis

TABLE 4. Summary of the cases of 155 patients with exercise-induced acute renal failure (ALPE)

	Number of cases described	Mean (range) or number of positive cases
Age (years)	150	21.7 ± 7.8 (10–54)
Sex	154	Male 143 (92.9%), Female 11
Prodrome (flu-like symptoms)	61	28 (45.9%)
Analgesic ingestion	68	23 (33.8%)
Nausea/vomiting	116	111 (95.7%)
Slight fever	62	47 (75.8%)
Hypertension	68	35 (51.5%)
Duration of loin pain (days)	43	5.2 ± 3.4 (1–14)
Initial serum creatinine (before urography) (mg/dl)	110	4.7 ± 2.8 (0.6–15)
Maximum serum creatinine (mg/dl)	138	6.0 ± 3.1 (1.2–15) Hemodialysis 29
Duration of renal dysfunction (days)	112	13.6 ± 9.0 (3–60)
Wedge-shaped contrast enhancement by CT	57	+53 (93.0%) –4
Duration of wedge-shaped lesions (h)	28	48.3 ± 25.8 (10–120)
Patchy lesions by MDP bone scan	28	+18 (64.3%) –10
Oliguria	126	24 (19.0%)
UOsm (mOsm/l)	23	283.9 ± 68.8 (170–408)
UNa (mEq/l)	28	46.7 ± 21.7 (14–99)
FENa (%)	51	2.0 ± 2.2 (0.07–12)
Myoglobinuria	91	0
Serum myoglobin (ng/ml) (Ratio to normal)	60	115.6 ± 123.6 (3.5–728) (1.6 ± 1.3 (1–7))
CPK (U/l) (Ratio to normal)	98	354.4 ± 486.8 (18–2863) (2.0 ± 1.7 (1–8.8))
Renal hypouricemia	133	76 (57.1%)
Recurrence of ALPE	155	31 (20.0%)

MDP, ^{99m}Tc-methylene diphosphonate

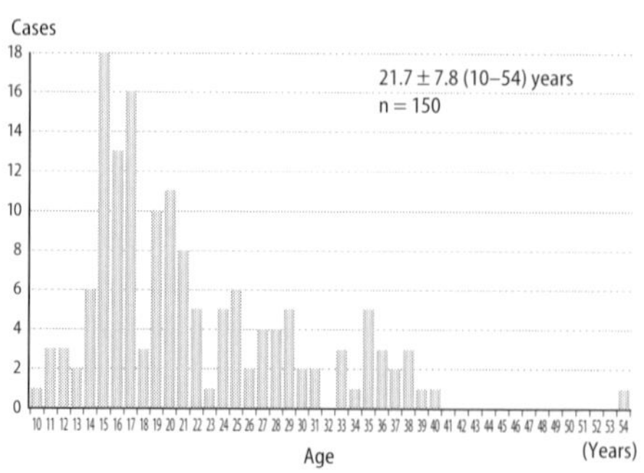

FIG. 46. Age distribution in 150 patients with ALPE. ALPE frequently develops at 14–25 years of age

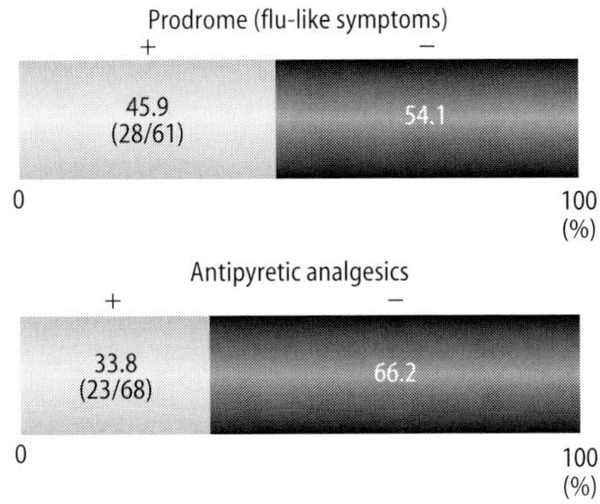

FIG. 47. Proportions of patients with a cold and those taking antipyretic analgesics before the onset of ALPE

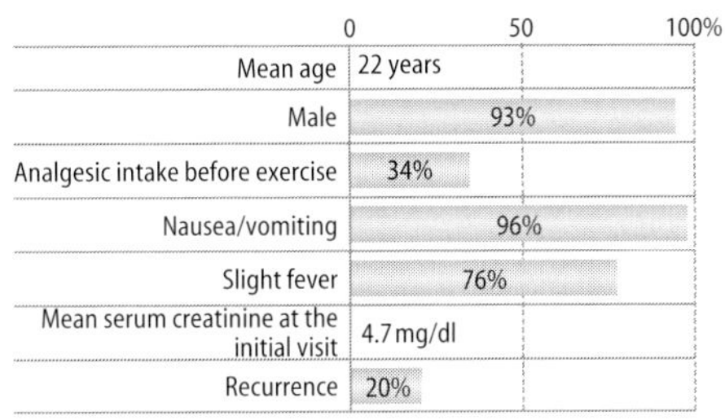

FIG. 48. Summary of 155 patients with ALPE

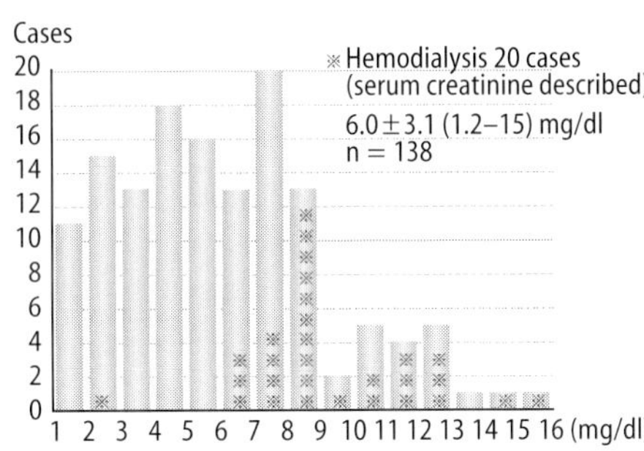

FIG. 49. Distribution of maximum serum creatinine levels in patients with ALPE. ※, patients who required hemodialysis

for all patients was good. However, 31 (20.0%) of 155 patients required dialysis therapy, or 29 (21.0%) of 138 patients for who serum creatinine levels were recorded required dialysis therapy.

Serum levels of creatine phosphokinase (CPK) (Fig. 50) were 100 mU/ml or less in 31 patients, and 300 mU/ml or more in 36 patients. The mean was 2.0 ± 1.7 times higher than the reference value. No values were more than 9 times higher than the reference value. However, minimal rhabdomyolysis was suggested.

The serum myoglobin level (Fig. 51) was 100 ng/ml or less in most patients (n = 42), and exceeded 300 ng/ml in only 4 patients. The mean was 1.6 ± 1.3 times higher than the reference value. No values were more than 7 times higher than the reference

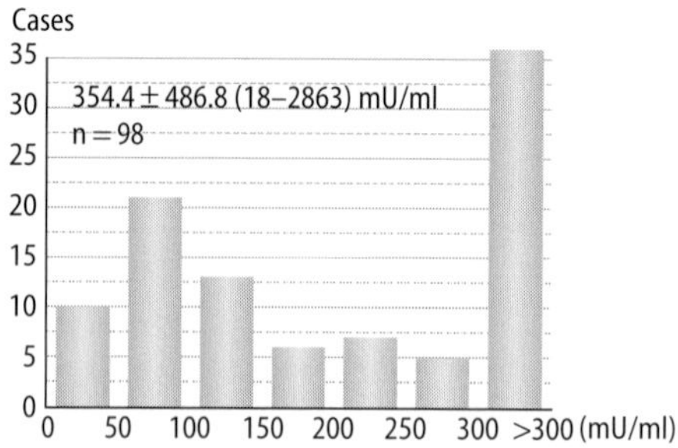

FIG. 50. Distribution of creatine phosphokinase (CPK) levels in patients with ALPE

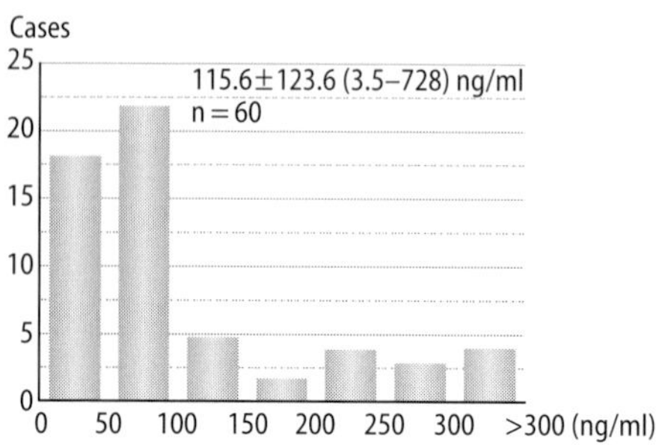

FIG. 51. Serum myoglobin levels in patients with ALPE

value. No patient showed myoglobinuria. In other words, the serum CPK and myoglobin levels in ALPE patients were normal or slightly increased. However, in none of these patients were these parameters more than 10–20 times higher than the reference values, which is different from the values found in myoglobinuric acute renal failure [11,137].

The urinalysis showed that there were no abnormalities in some patients, but mild proteinuria and hematuria were observed in others. UOsm was 284 ± 69 mOsm/l (n = 23), and UNa was 47 ± 22 mEq/l (n = 28). The mean values of FENa were 2.0 ± 2.2% and less than 1% in about 50% of patients, and 1% or more in the remaining patients.

3 Renal Hypouricemia

Renal hypouricemia was observed in 76 (57%) of the 133 patients in whom the serum levels of uric acid were recorded. Patients with a serum uric acid level of 2.0 mg/dl or less at baseline were regarded as having hypouricemia.

4 Imaging Findings (Wedge-Shaped Patchy Renal Ischemia)

Wedge-shaped contrast enhancement was detected in 53 (93%) of the 57 patients who underwent delayed computed tomography (CT) (Fig. 52). However, in the other 4 patients, CT was performed when the serum creatinine level was high.

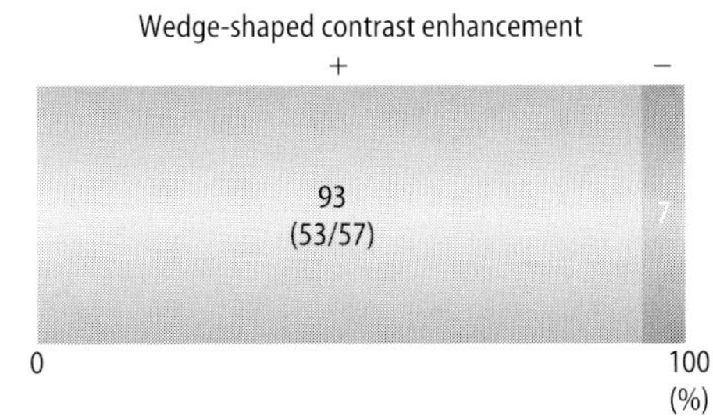

FIG. 52. Proportion of patients with wedge-shaped contrast enhancement in those who underwent delayed CT

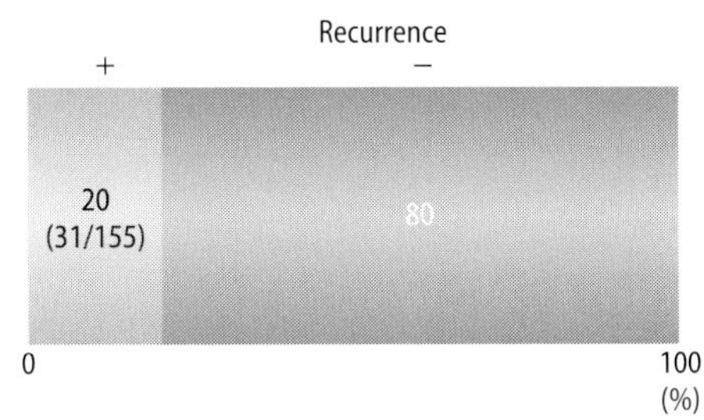

FIG. 53. Recurrence

5 Kidney Biopsy

In 54 patients, a kidney biopsy was performed 13.2 ± 8.9 days after onset ($n = 32$). In all patients, the findings suggested either acute tubular necrosis or its recovery phase. The underlying diseases included kidney diseases such as IgA nephropathy [138], minimal change nephrotic syndrome [139], autosomal dominant polycystic kidney disease (ADPKD) [140], and cystinuria [67].

6 Relapse

Relapse was detected in 31 (20%) of the 155 patients (Fig. 53). In one patient, 5 recurrent episodes were noted [117].

Chapter 7
Exercise

1 Type of Exercise

As shown in Fig. 54, the types of exercise taken by the patients consisted of a track race (a short-distance sprint such as a 200-m race), soccer, a swimming race, baseball, weightlifting, and a bicycle race, in all of which an intense power output per second or per minute is repeated. However, a single 100-m race was less likely to cause exercise-induced acute renal failure (ALPE). Several 200-m or 100-m races frequently caused ALPE. Repeated anaerobic exercise may be a risk factor.

The time of onset was often September or October, when many athletics meetings and sports festivals are held (Fig. 55).

2 Anaerobic Exercise

Anaerobic exercise (Table 5) is intense exercise requiring great muscle strength, such as sprinting and weightlifting. The activity is performed over a short period of time via explosive energy production/consumption [141–143]. A characteristic of such exercise is that can be performed via anaerobic glycolysis under a condition of oxygen deficiency. However, the duration of such exercise is limited to 1 min or less; it is impossible to continue anaerobic exercise for many hours. In anaerobic exercise it is type II muscle fibers (white muscle) that are mainly utilized.

TABLE 5. Aerobic and anaerobic exercise

	Aerobic exercise	Anaerobic exercise
Exercise, duration of exercise	Slow, long duration	Rapid, short duration (less than 1 min)
Type of exercise	Rapid walking, long-distance race, marathon, mountain climbing	Sprint, short-distance race, weightlifting
Mainly utilized muscle fibers	Type I muscle fibers	Type II muscle fibers
Energy source	ATP production due to oxidation of fatty acid and glucose	Stored ATP and ATP production from creatine phosphate and anaerobic glycolysis

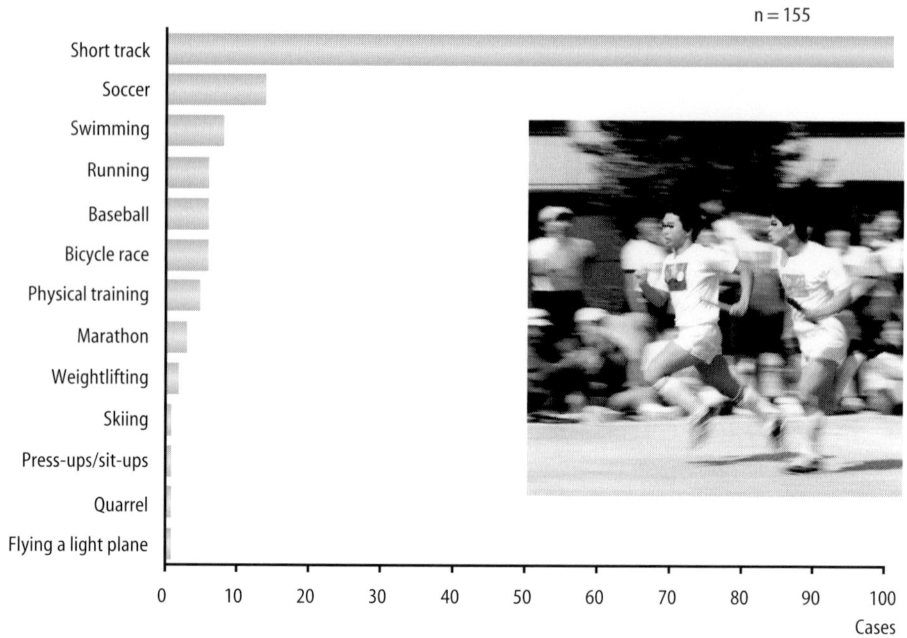

FIG. 54. Type of exercise causing ALPE. In most patients, anaerobic exercise was involved

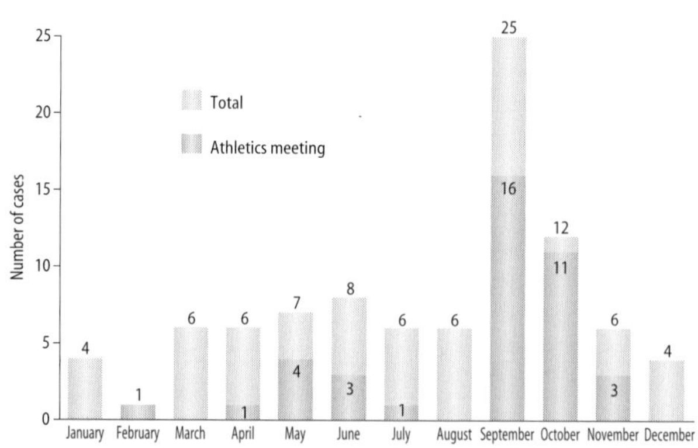

FIG. 55. Timing of ALPE development. The number of patients was highest in September, when many athletics meetings and sports festivals are held

TABLE 6. Types of muscle fibers

Type of muscle fiber	Type I Red muscle Aerobic exercise	Type II White muscle Anaerobic exercise
Glycogen	Small amount	Large amount
Enzyme activity of glycolysis	Small amount	Large amount
Enzyme activity of oxidation	High	Low
Mitochondria	Large amount	Small amount
Myoglobin	Large amount	Small amount

3 Involvement of Type II Muscle Fibers

Type II muscle fibers (white muscle, fast muscle) (Table 6) contribute to rapid muscle contraction by using energy obtained from stored ATP, and ATP production from creatine phosphate and anaerobic glycolysis of glycogen. However, the myoglobin content of these fibers is low [144,145], which may lead to less marked increases in serum myoglobin and creatine phosphokinase (CPK) in patients with ALPE.

Chapter 8
Loin Pain

1 Timing of Onset and Duration

In these patients, pain mainly developed 3–12 h (1–48 h) after exercise, and persisted for 1–14 days, with a mean of 5 days.

2 Sites and Features of Pain

Table 7 shows the sites and features of reported pain. Most patients complained of loin pain. However, some patients complained of abdominal pain. The grade of pain in our patients was severe in 10 of the 22 patients, making lying down, sleeping, and driving impossible.

Because of the severe pain, the physician (Patient 5) with exercise-induced acute renal failure (ALPE) made a self-diagnosis of acute pancreatitis. Initially, most patients are diagnosed as having ureteral stone, but some physicians diagnose "lumbar pain" or lumbar disc hernia.

TABLE 7. Sites and features of pain

Site of pain	Number of cases
Loin pain	103
Lumbar pain	23
Abdominal pain	28
Anterior chest pain	1
	155
Feature of pain	**Number of cases**
Rolling over due to acute severe pain	3
Cannot sleep at night	3
Cannot drive a car due to acute severe pain	2
Colicky	2

3 Mechanism Involved in Pain

The mechanism involved in the pain remains to be clarified. However, we speculate that it is vascular spasm-related pain, i.e., the involvement of renal angina, based on the following findings. In our experience, catheter end-related obstruction of the renal artery causes severe loin pain during selective renal angiography in patients undergoing dialysis, and one study reported that cerebrovascular spasm in the presence of subarachnoid hemorrhage persisted for 1 week in some patients. Acute tubular necrosis rarely induces renal swelling-related pain (nephralgia as a type of visceral pain), which may differ from the pain described above. The loin pain hematuria syndrome reported in the UK was related to renal infarction [146–148]. Loin pain in the presence of hemorrhagic fever with renal syndrome was associated with retroperitoneal edema [18]. These mechanisms differed from the mechanism involved in pain related to ALPE.

Chapter 9
Renal Hypouricemia

Risk factors for exercise-induced acute renal failure (ALPE) include anaerobic exercise, renal hypouricemia, administration of antipyretic analgesics for cold, and dehydration. We review renal hypouricemia here and in Chap.10.

1 Serum Creatinine and Uric Acid Levels

In 1990, we reported that 3 (23%) of 13 patients with ALPE had renal hypouricemia [3]. Previously, Erley et al. [28] had reported that patients with renal hypouricemia frequently developed acute renal failure. However, we were the first to report that these patients developed exercise-induced acute renal failure (ALPE) [3]. In our 3 patients with renal hypouricemia, the mean serum creatinine and uric acid levels in acute renal failure were 5.1 ± 2.6 mg/dl and 4.7 ± 1.7 mg/dl, respectively (Fig. 56). In the remaining 10 patients without renal hypouricemia, the mean serum creatinine and uric acid levels were 3.1 ± 1.6 mg/dl and 11.4 ± 4.2 mg/dl, respectively. In the recovery phase, these levels in the hypouricemia patients were 1.1 ± 0.3 mg/dl and 0.8 ± 0.2 mg/dl, respectively. The mean FEUA was 58.4 ± 18.7%. In the 10 patients without hypouricemia, the mean serum creatinine, uric acid, and FEUA values were 1.1 ± 0.1 mg/dl, 6.1 ± 1.2 mg/dl, and 7.8 ± 3.0%, respectively.

Previously, the disordered renal transport of uric acid in patients with renal hypouricemia had been explained by a 4-component model. In our review, 59% of the patients with ALPE and renal hypouricemia were classified as the presecretory reabsorption defect type, followed by the total defect in uric acid transport (no secretion and no reabsorption) and total reabsorption defect types (Table 8).

2 Comparison of Patients With and Without Renal Hypouricemia

Of the 155 cases of patients with ALPE collected from the literature, we examined the presence or absence of renal hypouricemia in 133 for whom the serum levels of uric acid were reported (Table 9). The mean ages in the renal hypouricemia and non-renal hypouricemia groups were 20.2 ± 7.4 years and 23.3 ± 8.4 years, respectively. In the

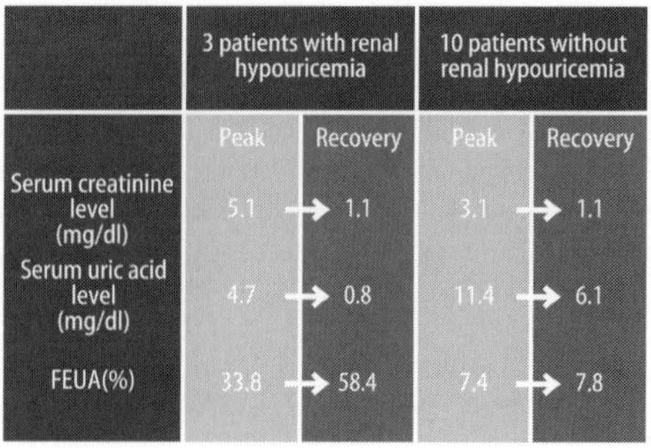

FIG. 56. Serum creatinine, uric acid, and FEUA values at the onset (peak) and recovery of ALPE in patients with and without renal hypouricemia

TABLE 8. Types of disordered renal uric acid transport in 76 patients with renal hypouricemia and ALPE

1. Presecretory reabsorption defect	29 (59.2%)
2. Total defect in uric acid transport (no secretion and no reabsorption)	10 (20.4%)
3. Total or subtotal reabsorption defect	8 (16.3%)
4. Postsecretory reabsorption defect	1 (2.0%)
5. Increased secretion	1 (2.0%)
6. Unknown or no description	27

TABLE 9. Comparison of ALPE patients with and without renal hypouricemia

	Renal hypouricemia	No renal hypouricemia	
n	76	57	
Age (years)	20.2 ± 7.4 (n = 75)	23.3 ± 8.4 (n = 57)	p = 0.0247
Male/female ratio	11.5:1	10.4:1	NS
Analgesic ingestion	2/16	14/42	NS
Prodrome (flu-like symptoms)	7/19	18/37	NS
Nausea/vomiting	57/58	42/45	NS
Slight fever	19/21	23/35	p = 0.0383
Duration of loin pain (days)	5.6 ± 4.3 (n = 17)	4.8 ± 2.8 (n = 24)	NS
Initial serum creatinine (mg/dl)	5.1 ± 2.8 (1.1–15) (n = 61)	4.0 ± 2.6 (0.6–11.3) (n = 42)	p = 0.0489
Maximum serum creatinine (mg/dl)	6.3 ± 2.9 (1.6–15) (n = 68)	5.6 ± 3.2 (1.2–14.1) (n = 54)	NS
Duration of renal dysfunction (days)	15.3 ± 9.0 (3–60) (n = 53)	12.4 ± 9.6 (3–60) (n = 44)	NS
Wedge-shaped lesions by CT scan	16/17	37/39	NS
Patchy lesion by MDP bone scan	4/7	12/19	NS
Oliguria	13/57	9/49	NS
Myoglobinuria	0/40	0/37	(NS)
Serum myoglobin (ng/ml)	126.4 ± 157.1 (n = 24)	120.0 ± 106.5 (n = 28)	NS
(Ratio to normal)	1.7 ± 1.4 (n = 28)	1.7 ± 1.3 (n = 31)	NS
CPK (U/l)	320.4 ± 471.2 (n = 42)	426.0 ± 522.5 (n = 46)	NS
(Ratio to normal)	1.8 ± 1.5 (n = 52)	2.3 ± 1.9 (n = 49)	NS
Recurrence of ALPE	23	6	p = 0.0064
Hypertension	20/39	12/25	NS

former group, the incidence of slight fever, serum creatinine level on the first visit, and recurrence rate were high. This renal hypouricemia group consisted of 76 patients (57%), and this percentage was markedly higher than that in our series (23%, 3/13). Furthermore, we calculated the incidence of ALPE in renal hypouricemia patients based on the incidence of renal hypouricemia in Japan and the proportion of patients with renal hypouricemia in ALPE patients. The incidence of ALPE in renal hypouricemia patients was approximately 50 times higher than that in non-renal hypouricemia patients.

We performed delayed CT after the administration of contrast medium in 11 patients with both ALPE and renal hypouricemia. In 10 of the 11 patients, patchy renal ischemia was noted [4], suggesting that renal ischemic conditions after anaerobic exercise were similar regardless of the presence or absence of renal hypouricemia.

3 Reasons for a High Incidence of ALPE in Patients with Renal Hypouricemia

A high incidence of ALPE was diagnosed in patients with renal hypouricemia because a uric acid transporter encoded by the SLC22A12 gene (uric acid transporter 1 (URAT1)) was identified in 2002 [149], a less marked increase in the serum uric acid level in the presence of acute renal failure facilitated diagnosis, the incidence of renal hypouricemia was high in Japan (0.15% [150] or 0.2%–0.6% [151]), and athletics meetings and sports festivals involving anaerobic exercise in the events are held as annual functions in schools, companies, and towns. These annual functions originated in an athletics meeting held at the Tokyo Navy Dormitory in 1874, where the main event was a short-distance sprint. Therefore, ALPE is a particularly important disorder in Japan.

4 Reason why Patients with Renal Hypouricemia Frequently Develop ALPE, and its Mechanism

4.1 Reason

It remains to be clarified why patients with renal hypouricemia frequently develop acute renal failure. The following hypothesis has been proposed. Oxidative stress is essential for the onset of ischemic acute renal failure. In the kidney, uric acid acts as a protective mechanism against oxidative stress. However, in patients with renal hypouricemia, a decrease in uric acid may allow exposure of the kidney to oxidative stress, causing ALPE [152,153].

4.2 Mechanism

The mechanism by which these patients develop ALPE also remains to be clarified. However, two hypotheses have been put forward, and active oxygen/renovascular spasm or tubular obstruction may be involved. One hypothesis is that patients with renal hypouricemia are exposed to active oxygen because the level of an active oxygen scavenger, uric acid, is reduced. Therefore, exercise may increase active oxygen, causing spasm of the interlobar/arcuate arteries. Furthermore, blood reperfusion may promote the production of active oxygen, causing ALPE. Recently, Perlstein et al. [154] reported that hyperuricemia inhibited angiotensin-related renovascular constriction. Therefore, anaerobic exercise may enhance angiotensin-related renovascular constriction in the presence of renal hypouricemia, causing patchy renal ischemia.

The other hypothesis is related to the fact that the reabsorption of uric acid is impaired in patients with renal hypouricemia. Even when exercise increases the serum uric acid level, uric acid is not reabsorbed, thus gradually increasing the tubular level of uric acid. In addition, exercise-related dehydration and urine acidification may result in tubular occlusion via the crystallization of uric acid, causing ALPE. The tubular events may be similar to the pathogenesis of acute uric acid nephropathy. Yeun and Hasbargen [59] supported this hypothesis. However, it remains controversial whether ALPE is associated with tubular obstruction due to uric acid crystals. The data do not support this hypothesis. Previously published case reports have shown the following findings. (1) Uric acid crystals were detected in the urinary sediment in the initial phase in only 3 of 76 patients with ALPE. (2) The histological findings within the first 10 days after onset in 9 of 28 patients who underwent kidney biopsy (mean interval from onset until kidney biopsy 11 $\pm$ 8 days) did not suggest acute uric acid nephropathy. However, there was no information on alcohol fixation for detecting uric acid crystals. (3) Patients with acute uric acid nephropathy are reported to show a UUA/Ucr value of 1.0 or more. However, the mean UUA/Ucr ratio was approximately 0.4 in our series (including patients without renal hypouricemia). (4) In our exercise load test, the glomerular filtration rate reduced after exercise in patients with a history of ALPE, and then FEUA increased (as described below). (5) In patients with severe ALPE requiring dialysis, wedge-shaped contrast enhancement was also observed in the recovery phase. (6) It is difficult to explain loin pain and wedge-shaped contrast enhancement by the hypothesis involving tubular occlusion.

In conclusion, intrarenal topical circulatory disorder or vascular spasm may develop in patients with renal hypouricemia, leading to acute renal failure.

Chapter 10
Gene Analysis of Uric Acid Transporter (URAT1)

1 URAT1 Gene Analysis in Patients with Renal Hypouricemia who Developed ALPE

In 7 patients with renal hypouricemia who developed exercise-induced acute renal failure (ALPE), gene analysis was performed to investigate URAT1 mutation [117,126,149,155] (Table 10, Cases 1–7). The W258X homozygote, W258X heterozygote, and W258X/Q297X compound heterozygote were detected in 5, 1, and 1 patients, respectively.

We encountered a father (Patient 18) and his son (Patient 21) with renal hypouricemia who both developed ALPE (Table 10, Cases 8 and 9). The W258X homozygote was not detected in either patient. The father showed the R90H homozygote, and his son showed the R90H/W258X compound heterozygote. The details of these two patients are given below [36] (Fig. 57).

Patient 18: a 41-year-old man (father, Patient 1 in Fig. 57)

On June 6, this patient developed severe loin pain after he participated in two 150-m sprints at a town athletics meeting. After 5 days, he was referred to the outpatient clinic of our department. His serum creatinine and uric acid levels and FEUA, were 2.9 mg/dl, 2.1 mg/dl, and 49.7%, respectively. His creatine phosphokinase (CPK) level was normal. When his serum creatinine level decreased to 1.58 mg/dl, a contrast medium was administered. A delayed computed tomography (CT) scan after 24 and 48 h confirmed patchy wedge-shaped contrast enhancement (Fig. 58). Under a diagnosis of ALPE, his body water balance (hydration) was controlled. In this patient, recovery was achieved 4 weeks after onset, and his serum creatinine and uric acid levels were then 1.0 mg/dl and 0.6 mg/dl, respectively. Furthermore, load tests with a uric acid reabsorption inhibitor (benzbromarone) and a uric acid excretion inhibitor (pyrazinamide) suggested presecretory reabsorption defect-related renal hypouricemia. A kidney biopsy 16 days after onset confirmed the recovery from acute tubular necrosis.

Patient 21: a 14-year-old boy (son, Patient 2 in Fig. 57)

This patient developed severe loin pain 3 h after he participated in two 400-m races, a mock cavalry battle, and a tug of war at an athletics meeting, and he attended a

Table 10. URAT1 (SLC22A12) mutation in patients with renal hypouricemia who developed ALPE

Case	Age (years)	Sex	Exercise	Loin pain	Serum uric acid (after recovery)	FEUA	URAT1 mutation	Literature
1	48	M	Exercise	No description	4.3 μg/ml	95%	W258X homozygote	Enomoto 2002[149)]
2	45	M	Strenuous exercise	Abdominal pain	0.8 mg/dl	46%	W258X homozygote	Tanaka 2003[117)]
3	42	M	Strenuous exercise	Back pain	1.0 mg/dl	65.7%	W258X homozygote	Tanaka 2003[117)]
4	No description	M	Exercise	No description	1.0 mg/dl	85.1%	W258X homozygote	Ichida 2004[155)]
5	No description	M	Exercise	No description	0.7 mg/dl	47.9%	W258X/Q297X compound heterozygote	Ichida 2004[155)]
6	No description	M	Exercise	No description	0.6 mg/dl	97.1%	W258X heterozygote	Ichida 2004[155)]
7	18	M	Strenuous exercise	Loin pain	0.9 mg/dl	50.1%	W258X homozygote	Nagaba 2004[126)]
8	41	M	150-m track race	Loin pain	0.6 mg/dl	67.0%	R90H homozygote	Ishikawa 2005[36)]
9	14	M	400-m track race	Loin pain	0.7 mg/dl	50.7%	R90H/W258X compound heterozygote	Ishikawa 2005[36)]

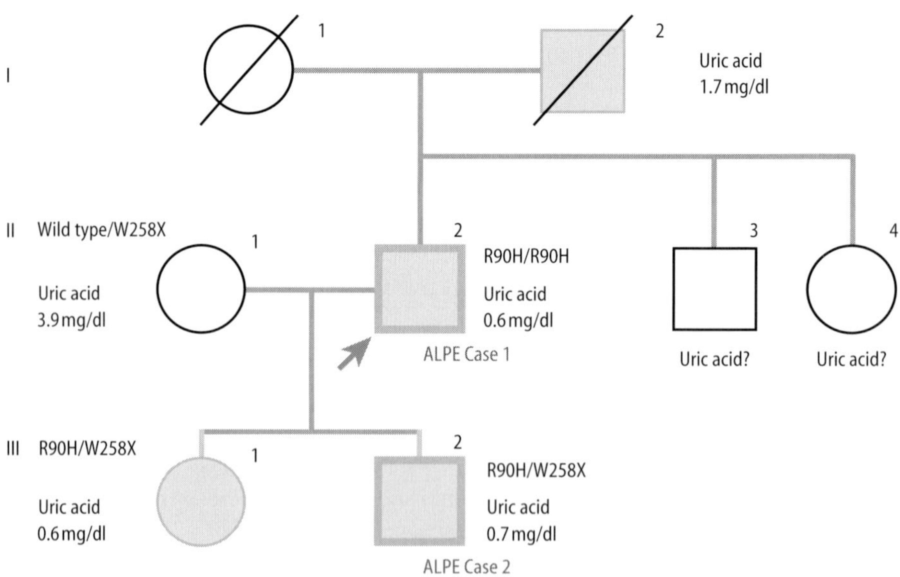

Fig. 57. Family tree of patients with renal hypouricemia who developed ALPE, and URAT1 (SLC22A12) gene analysis (From [36], with permission)

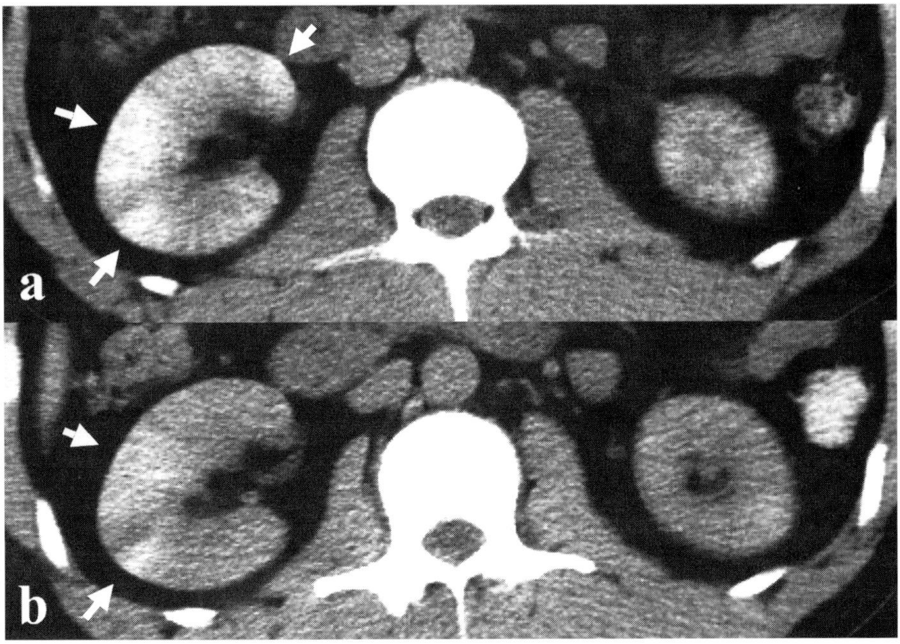

FIG. 58. Wedge-shaped contrast enhancement in Case 1 with ALPE in Fig. 57. **a**, 24h after; **b**, 48h after

local clinic. This occurred 5 years after his father had developed ALPE. His serum creatinine and CPK levels were 1.45mg/dl and 428U/l (reference value 44–212U/l), respectively. Under a diagnosis of muscular pain, a nonsteroidal anti-inflammatory drug (NSAID) was administered orally. However, after 3 days, he attended our hospital for loin pain and oliguria. His serum creatinine and uric acid levels were then 11.3mg/dl and 7.4mg/dl, respectively, and his FEUA was 65.7%, suggesting ALPE. This patient required 6 sessions of hemodialysis because of oliguria. After 4 weeks, both his serum creatinine and uric acid levels returned to 1.0mg/dl. In the recovery phase, 40ml contrast medium (iohexol) was administered. A delayed CT scan after 24h (serum creatinine 3.8mg/dl, Fig. 59) revealed multiple wedge-shaped contrast-enhanced areas. Furthermore, magnetic resonance imaging (MRI) 3min after the administration of gadolinium–diethylenetriaminopentoacetic acid (Gd–DTPA) (serum creatinine 1.54mg/dl) showed an inversion of the delayed CT findings described above (Fig. 59) and less marked wedge-shaped low signal intensity. In this patient, the effects of benzbromarone and pyrazinamide suggested renal hypouricemia related to presecretory reabsorption defect.

We analyzed the SLC22A12 uric acid transport gene (URAT1) in 4 members of his family. After informed consent was obtained, a DNA sequence analysis for URAT1 was determined (Fig. 60). We examined the SLC22A12 exon and exon/

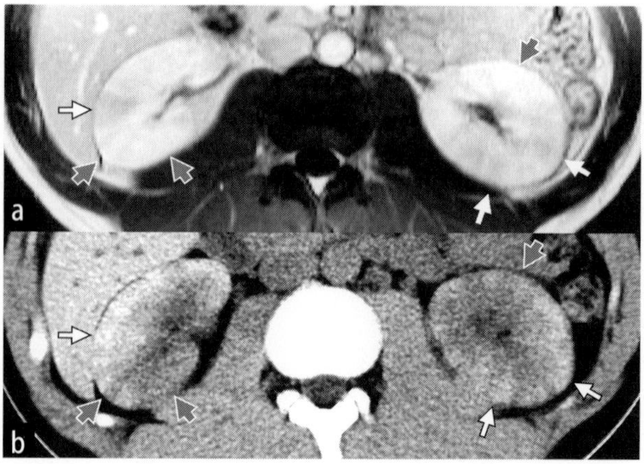

FIG. 59. Wedge-shaped contrast enhancement in Case 2 with ALPE in Fig. 57. **a**, MRI 3 min after the administration of Gd–DTPA (TR120, TE4.1/1). **b**, Delayed CT 24 h after the administration of contrast medium. These pictures are mirror images, as indicated by the *arrows* (From [36], with permission)

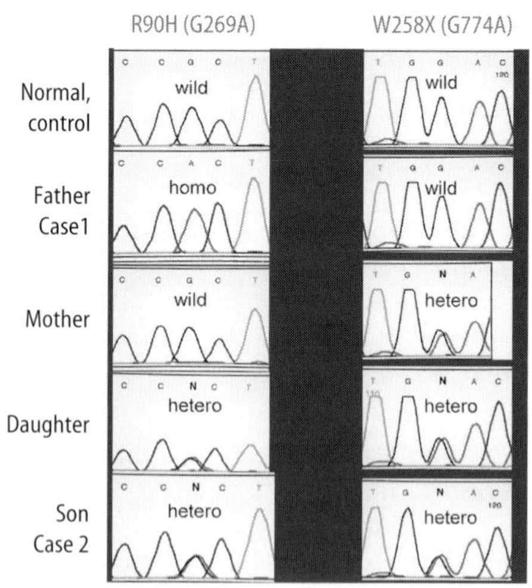

FIG. 60. Analysis of R90H (G269A) and W258X (G774A) by direct DNA sequencing in a family with renal hypouricemia

intron border areas using genomic DNA. As shown in Fig. 57, this patient's father had the R90H homozygote, and the patient had the R90H/W258X compound heterozygote. The patient's mother had the W258X heterozygote, showing a normal serum uric acid level. Her daughter had the R90H/W258X compound heterozygote involved in renal hypouricemia [36]. However, she did not have a history of ALPE.

Chapter 11
Risk Factors Other than Renal Hypouricemia

1 Exercise in the Presence of a Cold

At the onset of exercise-induced acute renal failure (ALPE), a slight fever was often observed, and most patients were positive for C-reactive protein (CRP). After considering the possibility of viral infection-associated ALPE, we investigated changes in the titers of various virus antibodies at onset and in the recovery phase. However, there were no significant changes.

2 Administration of Antipyretic Analgesics Before Exercise

In 34% of patients, anaerobic exercise after taking analgesic agents for a cold induced ALPE. The oral administration of nonsteroidal anti-inflammatory drugs (NSAIDs) may be a risk factor.

3 Exercise in the Presence of Dehydration

Dehydration is a risk factor for all types of acute renal failure. It promotes the onset of ALPE, but may not be an important factor. The significance of dehydration in the pathogenesis of ALPE remains to be clarified.

Chapter 12 Etiology/Pathogenesis

1 Hypothesis About the Development of Exercise-Induced Acute Renal Failure (ALPE)

The pathogenesis of ALPE remains to be clarified. However, we propose the following hypothesis [4] (Fig. 61). Initially, anaerobic exercise such as a sprint may cause anaerobic glycolysis disorder of type II muscle fibers. Subsequently, adenosine 5′-triphosphate (ATP) deficiency may result in muscular injury. As a result, renal vasoconstrictive factors other than myoglobin may be released, promoting renovascular spasm at the interlobar/arcuate artery levels. However, for some reason, the grade of spasm may differ from branch to branch. The vascular spasm may induce acute tubular necrosis without increases in creatine phosphokinase (CPK) and serum myoglobin on the one hand, and renal angina with loin pain on the other. Risk factors for ALPE include renal hypouricemia, analgesic agents, and dehydration. However, vasoconstrictive factors remain to be clarified, and the involvement of muscle-derived substances and active oxygen is assumed. Furthermore, it is unclear why the grade of vascular spasm differs among the renal arterial branches, and at present there is no hypothesis to explain this.

2 Investigation of Serum-Specific Markers (SDS–PAGE, Proteomics)

In order to clarify the vasoconstrictive factors, sodium dodecyl sulfate polyacrylamide gel electrophoresis (SDS–PAGE) was carried out in the initial phase of our study. In the patients with myoglobinuric acute renal failure, myoglobin bands were detected. However, there were no ALPE-specific bands (Fig. 62).

We carried out proteomic analysis using a surface-enhanced laser desorption/ionization time-of-flight mass spectrometry (SELDI–TOF–MS) and ProteinChips, which facilitate the analysis of low molecular weight proteins (Ishikawa, unpublished results, 2005). In the ALPE group, 18 marker candidates were found (molecular weight 3.5 KDa/4.3 KDa (Fig. 63)) in whom the relative intensity was higher than in the myoglobinuric acute renal failure and normal groups. We performed hierarchical clustering analysis by combining these marker candidates. In the ALPE group, the pattern differed from those in the myoglobinuric acute renal failure and normal groups (Fig. 64). However, no ALPE-specific single biomarker was found.

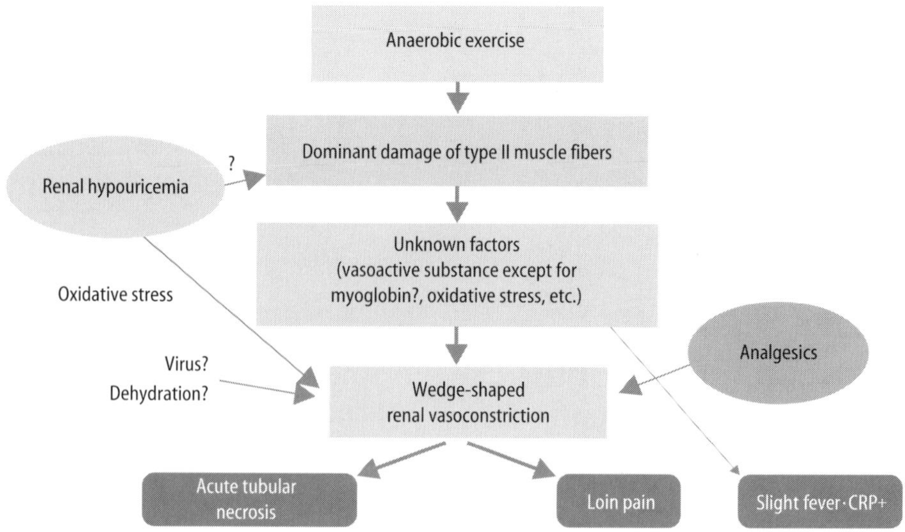

Fig. 61. Pathogenesis of ALPE (hypothesis)

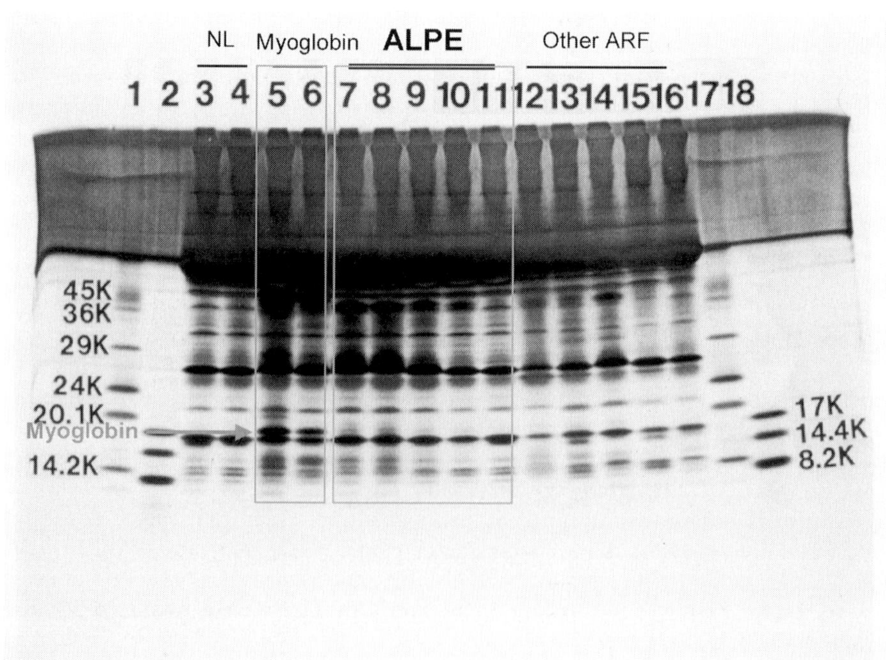

Fig. 62. SDS–PAGE in normal controls and in patients with myoglobinuric acute renal failure, ALPE, or acute renal failure related to other etiologies. There were no bands which were specific to ALPE. *ARF*, acute renal failure

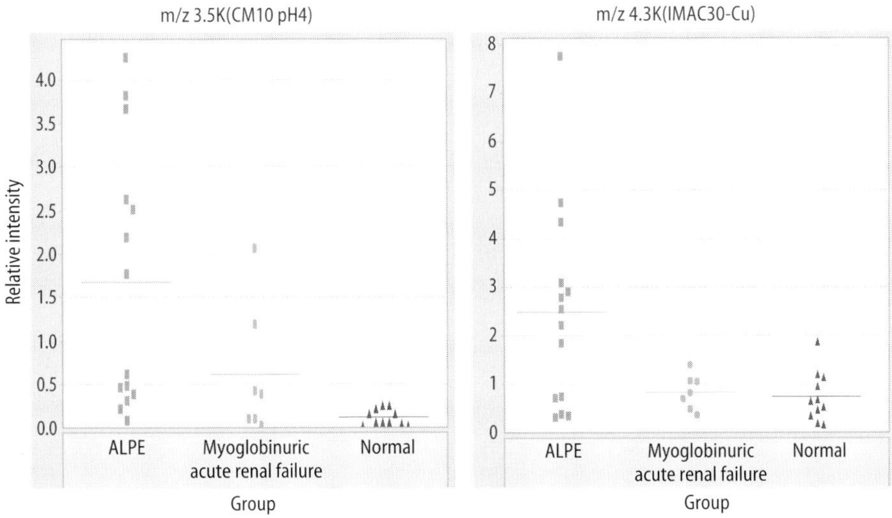

FIG. 63. Single marker analysis with surface-enhanced laser desorption/ionization time-of-flight mass spectrometry (SELDI–TOF–MS) in the ALPE, myoglobinuric acute renal failure, and normal groups. In the ALPE group, the relative intensity of a 3.5 KDa/4.3 KDa peptide was higher than that in the other groups

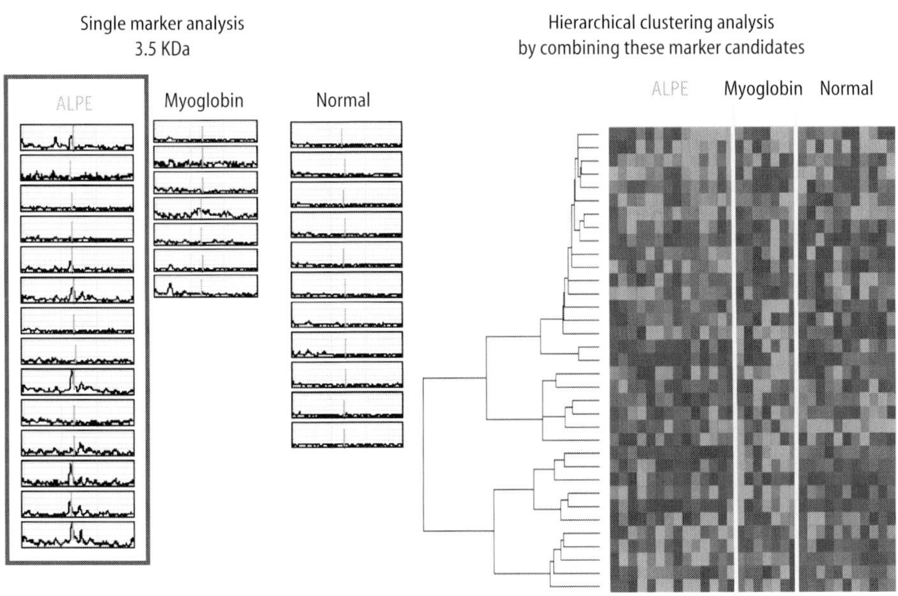

FIG. 64. Proteomic analysis with a SELDI–TOF–MS. In single marker analysis (*left*), the relative intensity of the 3.5 KDa peptide was high in the ALPE group. In the hierarchical clustering analysis with marker candidates, the heat map in the ALPE group differed from those in the myoglobinuric acute renal failure and normal groups

If several candidates are purified and identified in the future, some ALPE-specific markers may be found. However, the pathogenesis of patchy renovascular spasm may involve several factors, not just a single factor.

3 Investigation of Oxidative Stress Markers

Oxidative stress plays an important role in the onset of ischemic acute renal failure [156,157]. However, it is unclear whether oxidative stress is involved in the onset of ALPE. To investigate changes in oxidative stress, markers such as 8-isoprostane and NO*x* are used. In particular, 8-isoprostane is produced by prostaglandin in the presence of oxidative stress, and is considered to be a useful marker [158]. We measured 8-isoprostane as a marker, and investigated changes in oxidative stress using urine samples from patients with ALPE. In these patients, there was no increase in urinary 8-isoprostane even when their serum creatinine level was high. In the recovery phase, there was a transient increase (Fig. 65); there was no increase in oxidative stress, and the involvement of oxidative stress in the pathogenesis of ALPE has not been demonstrated.

4 Exercise Load Tests

Test 1

We enrolled five members of the Kanazawa Medical University Soccer Team (including one member with a history of ALPE) in order to examine changes in serum creatinine, serum myoglobin, and CPK before and after a match. There were no differences in the levels of change in these three parameters regardless of the presence or absence of a history of ALPE (Fig. 66). We did not investigate creatinine clearance.

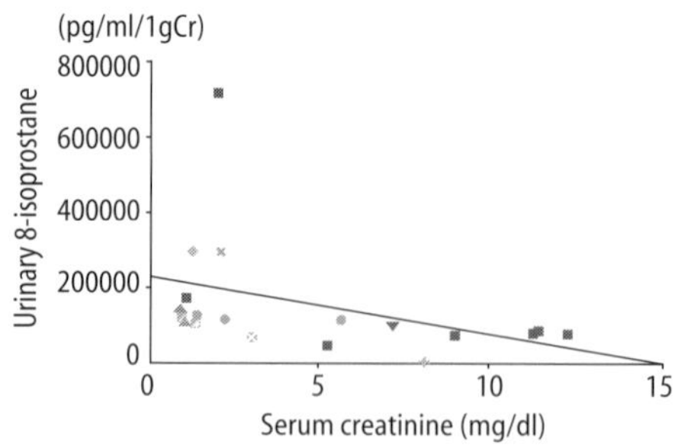

FIG. 65. Relationship between urinary 8-isoprostane and serum creatinine levels. In the initial phase, when the serum creatinine level was high, there was no increase in urinary 8-isoprostane. In the recovery phase, the urinary 8-isoprostane level increased

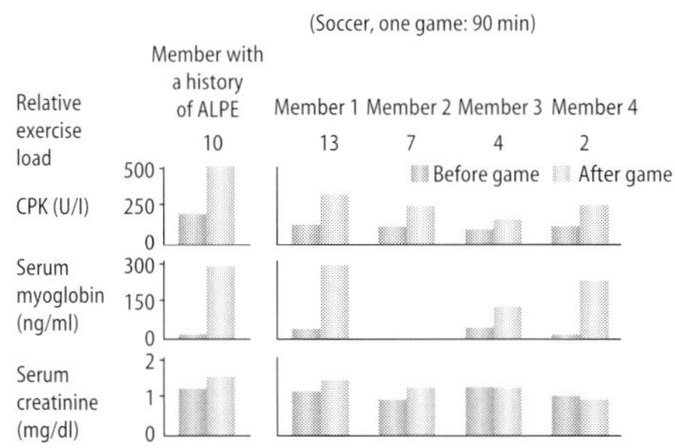

FIG. 66. Changes in CPK, serum myoglobin, and serum creatinine in the university soccer team members (including one member with a history of ALPE) before and after a soccer game. The increase in serum creatinine in the patient with a history of ALPE was not marked

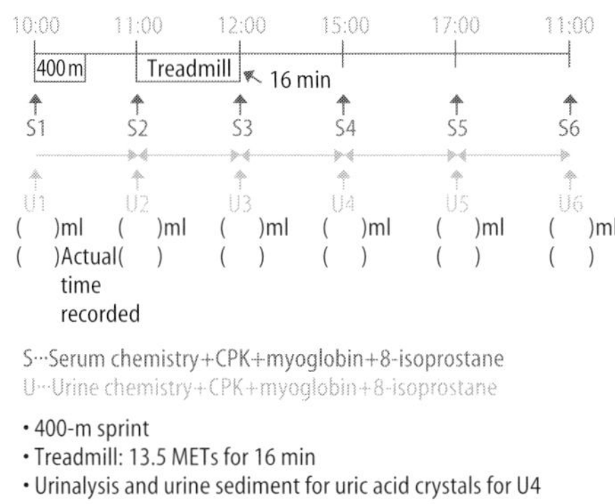

FIG. 67. Exercise load protocol. An anaerobic exercise load test was performed first, followed by an aerobic exercise load test

Test 2

We selected one renal hypouricemia patient with a history of ALPE and one healthy adult (control) without a history of ALPE, and measured creatinine clearance, FEUA, and oxidative stress markers (urinary 8-isoprostane and NO*x*) after anaerobic and aerobic exercise load tests (a 400-m race, 16 min on a treadmill, Bruce method, 13.5 metabolic equivalents (METs)) (Fig. 67). In the hypouricemia patient, (a) exercise reduced creatinine clearance (Fig. 68), (b) FEUA increased 5 h after the exercise load test (Fig. 69), (c) the urinary 8-isoprostane level increased slightly 6–25 h after the exercise load test, although there were no marked differences compared with the control values (Fig. 70), and (d) the urinary NO*x* level increased 2 and 5 h after the exercise load test (Fig. 71). Thus, we found that exercise reduced creatinine clearance in the renal hypouricemia patient with a history of ALPE, but there was no marked influence of oxidative stress.

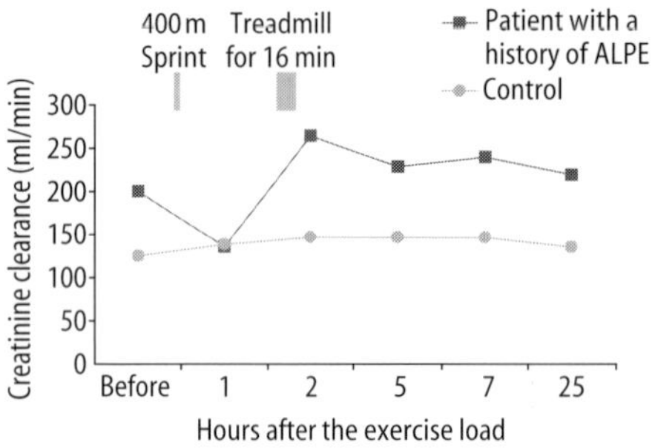

FIG. 68. Exercise loading and creatinine clearance. In the exercise loading protocol described in Fig. 67, creatinine clearance after anaerobic exercise was reduced in a patient with a history of ALPE

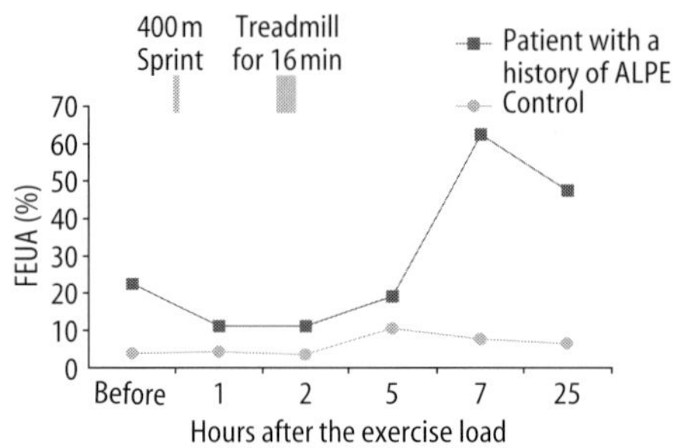

FIG. 69. Exercise loading and FEUA. In a patient with a history of ALPE, FEUA was reduced after exercise, but increased again 7–25 h later

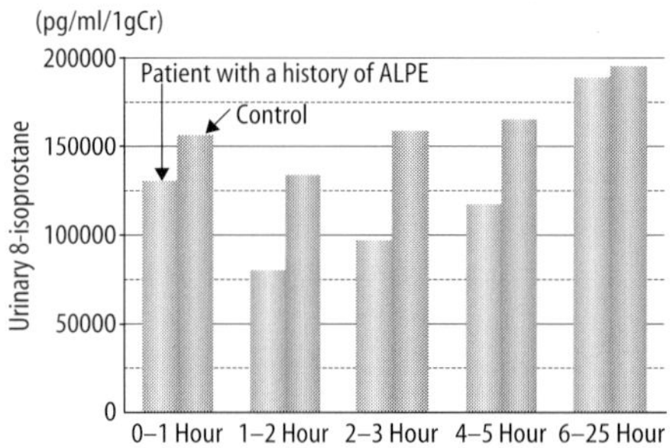

FIG. 70. Exercise loading and urinary 8-isoprostane levels. There were no marked differences in the changes in urinary 8-isoprostane between a patient with a history of ALPE and the control

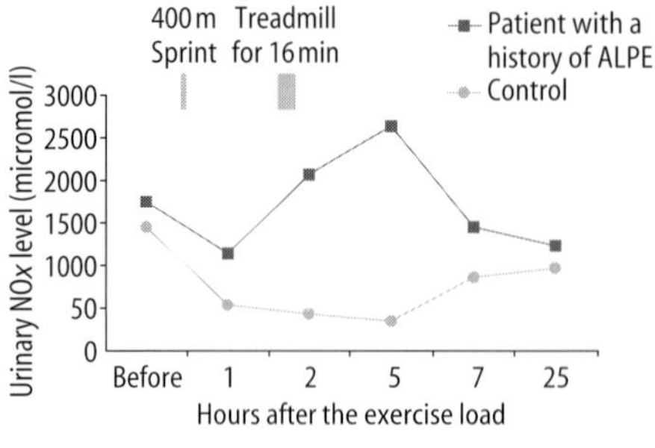

FIG. 71. Exercise loading and levels of urinary stable metabolites of NO (NOx). The changes in urinary NOx after exercise differed between a patient with a history of ALPE and the control

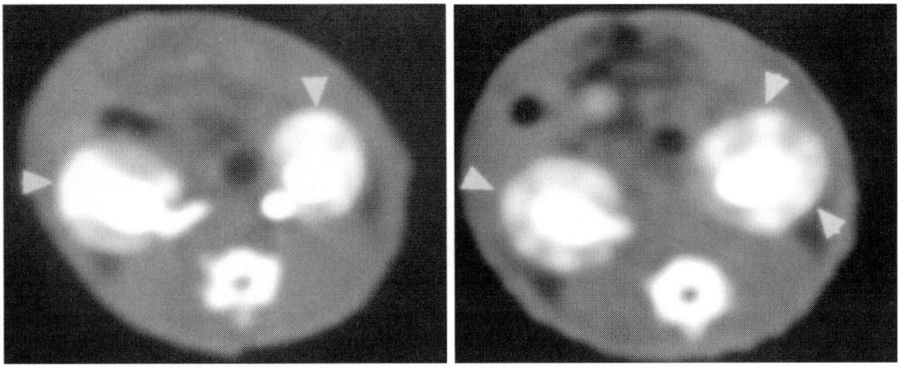

Fig. 72. Wedge-shaped contrast enhancement after the administration of vasopressin in an animal model

5 Preparation of Wedge-Shaped Patchy Renal Ischemia in an Animal Experiment

To prepare an ALPE model, rats were made to exercise in a cistern after the administration of a nonsteroidal anti-inflammatory drug (NSAID). However, ALPE did not develop. To obtain wedge-shaped contrast enhancement in rats, various vasoactive agents were employed. After the administration of endothelin, angiotensin, or epinephrine, only diffuse contrast enhancement was achieved. However, after the administration of vasopressin at 50 U/kg (a dose for achieving hemostasis for esophageal varices in humans), patchy wedge-shaped contrast enhancement was achieved [159] (Fig. 72). Vasoactive agents such as vasopressin may be involved in renovascular spasm.

6 Verification of Hypotheses

6.1 Does ALPE develop via the release of a renal vasoconstricting substance by type II muscle fibers?

Some studies have suggested that a vasoconstrictive substance other than myoglobin is released by muscles in the presence of rhabdomyolysis [160,161], although no vasoconstrictive substance has been identified by analysis with a SELDI–TOF–MS. However, patients with renal hypouricemia may be sensitive to vasoactive substances (such as angiotensin), and develop vascular spasm rather frequently. In an animal experiment, imaging after the administration of vasopressin showed patchy wedge-shaped contrast enhancement in the kidney. In addition, in some patients with ALPE, ischemia was observed not only in the kidney but also in other organs, suggesting concurrent vascular spasm in the intestinal tract, liver [43], and brain (cerebral infarction) [69]. These findings suggest that vasoconstrictive factors are involved in the onset of ALPE. However, the details remain to be clarified.

6.2 Involvement of active oxygen and various vasoactive substances

Exercise increases the levels of active oxygen and vasoactive substances such as endothelin, vasopressin, and catecholamines, and reduces the level of nitric oxide (NO). In this study, we investigated whether active oxygen is involved in the pathogenesis of ALPE. However, the results of measurements of 8-isoprostane and NO*x* did not suggest the involvement of active oxygen. Many patients with ALPE showed slight fever and an increase in C-reactive protein (CRP), although the association of these findings with the disorder was unclear. This suggests the involvement of inflammation and cytokines in the onset of ALPE. However, viral infection is ruled out. All possible mechanisms should be thoroughly investigated.

6.3 Why does vascular spasm persist for a long period?

We speculate that ischemia induces changes in the tubulo-interstitium by such factors as oxidative stress, apoptosis, an increase in intracellular Ca, complement activation, ICAM-1 expression, and inflammation, in a region controlled by the blood vessels, thereby influencing the blood vessels and prolonging vascular spasm. Coronary spasm persists for 15 min, and cerebrovascular spasm in the presence of subarachnoid hemorrhage persists for a week in some patients. Therefore, renovascular spasm may persist for a long period.

Chapter 13
Diagnosis

1 Initially Suspected Disorders

At the Emergency Outpatient Unit, most patients were initially diagnosed as having ureteral stone, or acute gastroenteritis based on vomiting/slight fever, or acute pancreatitis, lumbar pain, muscular pain, or lumbar disc hernia based on severe pain (Fig. 73).

2 Diagnosis of ALPE

In patients complaining of severe loin pain and nausea/vomiting after a sprint in an athletics meeting, a differential diagnosis of exercise-induced acute renal failure (ALPE) should be suggested, considering the risk of ALPE. In particular, this disorder must be considered first in patients with a history of ALPE. In the presence of ALPE, the serum creatinine level increases slightly a few hours after onset. However, neither myoglobinuria nor creatine phosphokinase (CPK) elevation is noted, which is different from what is usually found with rhabdomyolysis. When the serum uric acid level is normal or below the normal range despite an increase in the serum creatinine level, ALPE complicated by renal hypouricemia should be considered. In particular, this disorder may frequently recur when familial renal hypouricemia or a history of post-exercise loin pain is present.

3 Differentiation of ALPE from Myoglobinuric Acute Renal Failure

We compared ALPE (non-myoglobinuric acute renal failure) with myoglobinuric acute renal failure (Table 11).

ALPE frequently developed after anaerobic exercise, and caused severe loin pain, nausea/vomiting, and slight fever without dark urine. Furthermore, the serum myoglobin and CPK levels were normal or slightly increased, and delayed computed tomography (CT) showed wedge-shaped contrast enhancement.

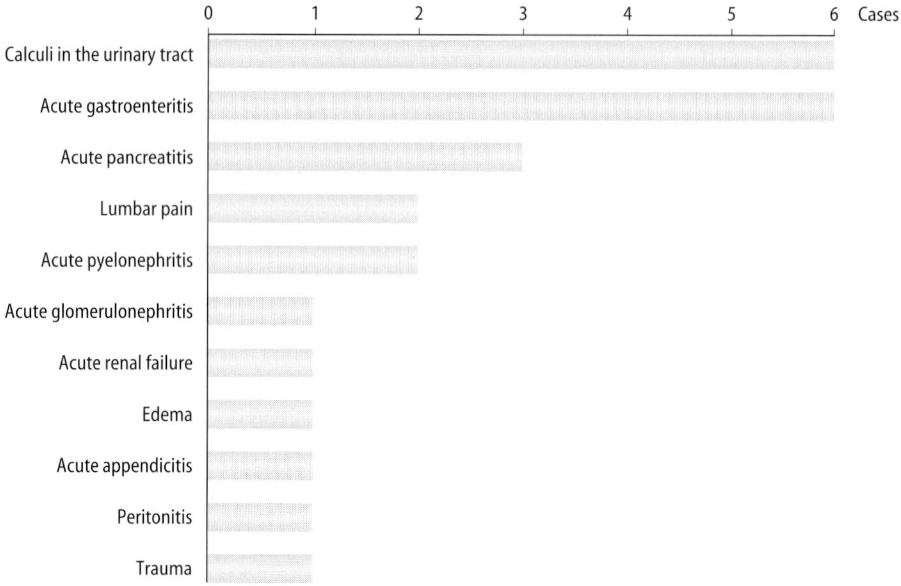

FIG. 73. Disorders suspected on the first visit to an outpatient department (in patients for whom the disorder was described)

TABLE 11. Differential diagnosis of exercise-induced acute renal failure (ALPE) from myoglobinuric acute renal failure

	Exercise-induced acute renal failure (ALPE)	Myoglobinuric acute renal failure
Extent of exercise	+	+++
Type of exercise	Anaerobic (track race, swimming)	Aerobic (marathon, mountain climbing)
Urine volume	Nonoliguric	Oliguric
Dark urine	–	+++
Loin pain	+++	– ~ +
Nausea, vomiting, slight fever	++	+
Dehydration	+	+++
Serum myoglobin, CPK	Normal or slightly increased	↑↑↑
Delayed CT scan after administration of contrast medium	Patchy wedge-shaped enhancement	Diffuse enhancement

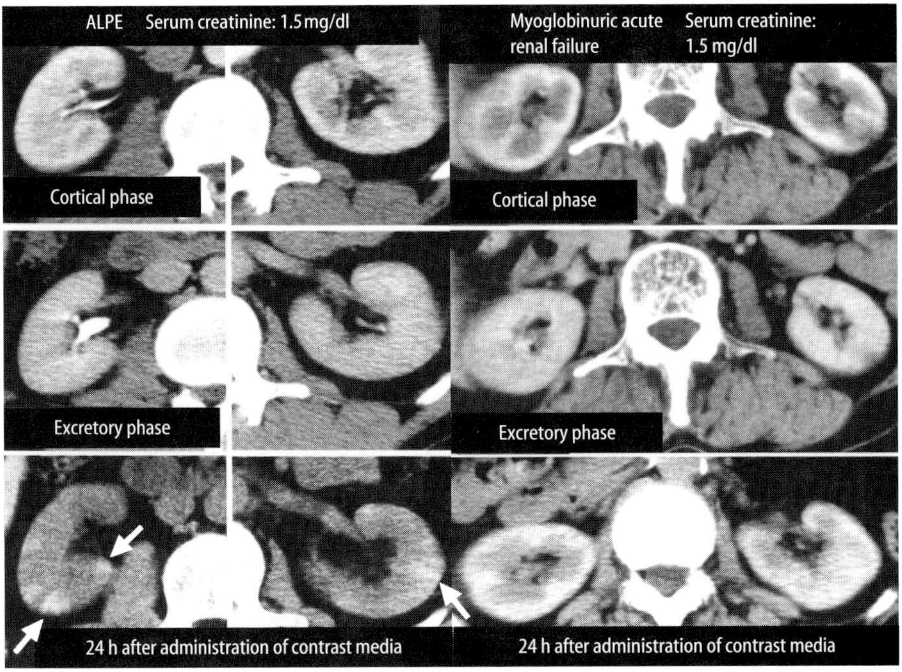

FIG. 74. Delayed CT in a patient with ALPE and a patient with myoglobinuric acute renal failure with a serum creatinine level of 1.5 mg/dl. In the patient with ALPE, wedge-shaped contrast enhancement was observed 24 h after the administration of a contrast medium. However, wedge-shaped contrast enhancement could not be confirmed in the cortical phase 20–40 s after the administration, or in the excretory phase 3 min after the administration (see Fig. 17). The patient with myoglobinuric acute renal failure showed diffuse contrast enhancement

Myoglobinuric acute renal failure developed after continued strenuous exercise. Marked muscular destruction (rhabdomyolysis) resulted in dark urine. However, there was no pain, and dehydration was marked. The CPK level showed a 10- to 20-fold increase compared with the reference value. Delayed CT showed diffuse contrast enhancement (Fig. 74).

In the patients with ALPE, bone scans showed no muscular uptake of methylene diphosphonate (MDP). However, upper/lower limb muscle uptake of MDP was found in the patients with myoglobinuric acute renal failure (Fig. 75).

As shown in Fig. 76, exercise-related acute renal failure is classified into two types: myoglobinuric acute renal failure and non-myoglobinuric acute renal failure. The latter is represented by ALPE. The grade of rhabdomyolysis and the type/grade of muscle fibers affected are shown in Fig. 76. Pathogenetic factors for ALPE should be investigated in the future.

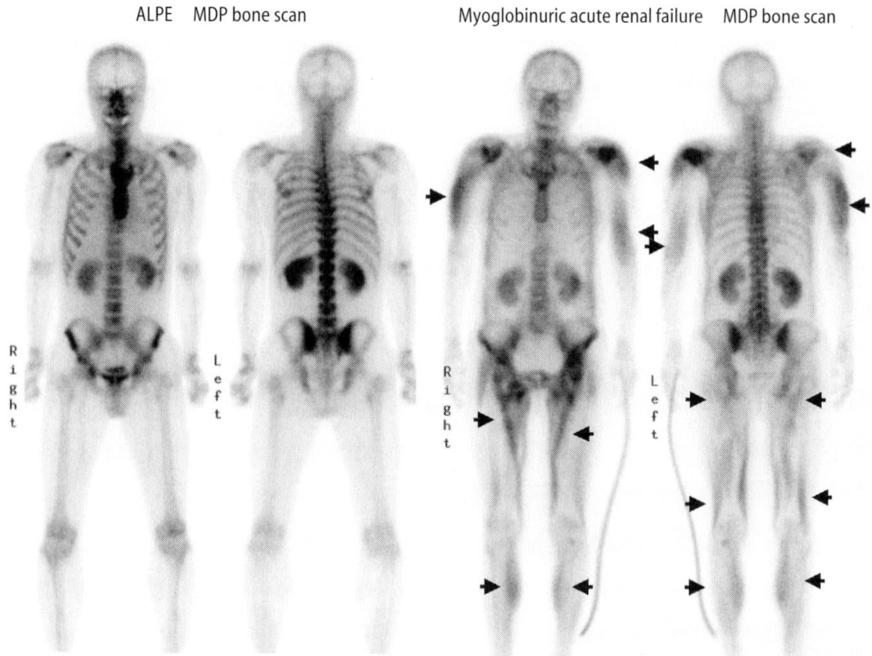

FIG. 75. Bone scan with MDP. In a patient with ALPE (*left*), there was no muscular uptake of MDP. However, muscular accumulation of MDP (*arrows*) was observed in a patient with myoglobinuric acute renal failure (*right*). In the ALPE patient, it was impossible to evaluate the presence or absence of patchy accumulation in the kidney

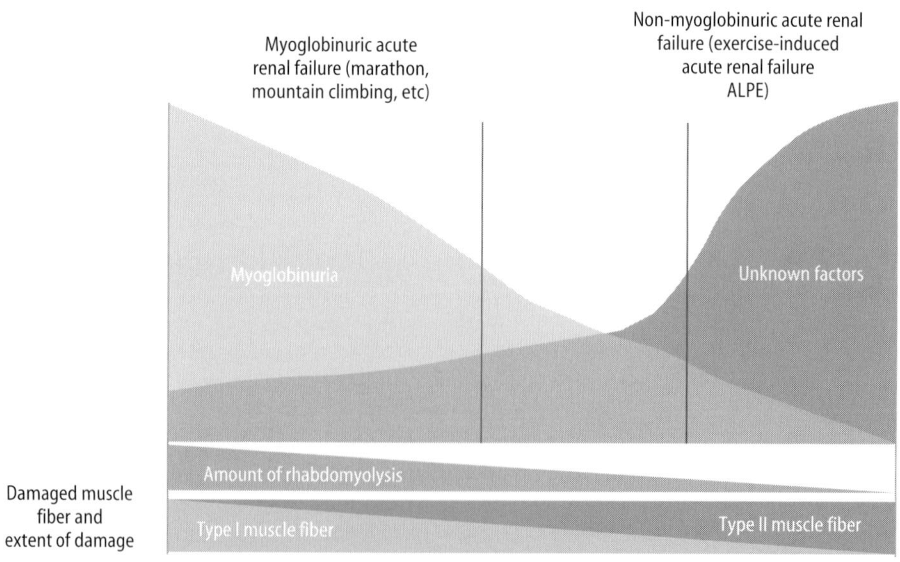

FIG. 76. Comparison of the pathogenesis between myoglobinuric acute renal failure and non-myoglobinuric acute renal failure represented by ALPE (hypothesis)

4 Necessity of Visualizing Wedge-Shaped Patchy Renal Ischemia

In the patients with ALPE, plain CT of the kidney (delayed CT) a few hours, 24 h, and 48 h after the administration of 40 ml contrast medium showed wedge-shaped contrast enhancement. When physicians hesitate to administer a contrast medium, patchy accumulation can be sometimes detected by magnetic resonance imaging (MRI) with gadolinium-diethylenetriaminopentoacetic acid (Gd-DTPA), bone scan with MDP, or ultrasonography with Levovist.

In addition to ALPE, mild acute renal failure, including dehydration, acute pyelonephritis, and renal pelvic tumors, is visualized as wedge-shaped contrast enhancement [15]. However, acute pyelonephritis and renal pelvic tumors are visualized as unilateral lesions, whereas ALPE is visualized as a bilateral lesion; therefore, differentiation is possible. For a definitive diagnosis, the presence of patchy contrast enhancement must be demonstrated when the serum creatinine level is in the range from 1.2 to 3.5 mg/dl. However, as described above, a definitive diagnosis is not always necessary in clinical practice.

Chapter 14
Treatment

1 Treatment

Treatment should be selected based on the grade of kidney dysfunction. In deciding on conservative therapy, hydration must be controlled. Hydration is normalized according to the presence or absence of overhydration and dehydration, although dehydration is rare. When oliguria, hyperpotassemia, and uremia are observed (21% of the patients), dialysis therapy should be considered according to the indication for dialysis therapy in acute tubular necrosis.

2 Precautions

As nonsteroidal anti-inflammatory drugs (NSAIDs) exacerbate ALPE, the administration of NSAIDs should be avoided even after onset. When patients require analgesic agents, synthetic opioid agonist/antagonist analgesics (pentazocine hydrochloride or buprenorphine hydrochloride) should be administered.

Chapter 15
Disease Course and Prognosis

1 Interval Required Until Improvement in Kidney Function

In our experience, the mean interval until the normalization of serum creatinine was 3 weeks.

2 Prognosis: Patients Undergoing Hemodialysis

This disorder shows a good prognosis, involving spontaneous recovery in most patients [4]. However, 29 (21.0%) of 138 patients required dialysis therapy owing to severe acute renal failure. No patient died in our series or in the literature consulted.

Chapter 16
Prevention

1 Preventive Methods

Methods of preventing exercise-induced acute renal failure (ALPE) and relapse have not been established as the etiology and pathogenesis of ALPE remain to be clarified. However, the following points are important.

1. Sprinting in an athletics meeting should be avoided if the athlete has a cold.
2. Nonsteroidal anti-inflammatory drugs (NSAIDs) should not be taken before exercise.
3. Exercise should be avoided in conditions of high temperature or humidity, and suitable preparatory exercise must be performed.
4. Repeated anaerobic exercise should be avoided.
5. The prevention of dehydration is essential (water supplementation, no exercise after drinking alcohol).
6. ALPE frequently develops and recurs in patients with renal hypouricemia, and caution is needed. When a relapse is suspected, patients should immediately consult a hospital without taking analgesic agents (NSAIDs). In particular, caution is needed when the patient's base-line serum uric acid level is 1.0 mg/dl or less.

Some investigators have recommended that antioxidants (allopurinol, vitamin C, vitamin E) are taken for 5 days prior to exercise in order to prevent ALPE. However, their effects are unclear.

2 Precautions for Elementary and Junior/Senior High Schools

If a renal hypouricemia patient with a serum uric acid level of 1.0 mg/dl or less wishes to join an athletics sports team (short track sprint) at school, a physician should instruct them to change to other activities. If a patient participates in a track event at an athletics meeting, a physician should instruct them to comply with the preventive methods described above.

Chapter 17
Conclusions

1. Exercise-induced acute renal failure (ALPE) frequently develops in young healthy males after repeated anaerobic exercise such as a 200-m race. The recurrence rate is high.

2. The risk of ALPE is high in patients with renal hypouricemia, and in those who have a cold and take antipyretic analgesics before exercise.

3. Severe loin pain persists for 5 days (mean). Because of the pain, patients are often misdiagnosed as having ureteral stone.

4. Plain computed tomography (CT) after the administration of contrast medium (delayed CT) shows wedge-shaped contrast enhancement in the bilateral kidneys, which persists for 1–3 days.

5. Many patients have non-oliguric acute renal failure, with a good prognosis. However, some patients require dialysis. For treatment, hydration must be controlled, and nonsteroidal anti-inflammatory drugs (NSAIDs) should be avoided if possible. When oliguria is observed, dialysis therapy should be performed, as described for acute tubular necrosis.

ALPE is different from exertional rhabdomyolysis (myoglobinuric acute renal failure).

Diagnosis and treatment should be performed with reference to the findings described above.

Postscript

We have reviewed the cases of patients with exercise-induced acute renal failure (ALPE) who we have encountered since 1979, when we treated the first patient in our series.

We are able to identify the presence of this disorder, and summarize the diagnosis and treatment because (a) we had personal contact with the patients, (b) we had previous knowledge of the hemodynamics of acute renal failure, (c) we had been carrying out animal experiments into glycerol-induced acute renal failure (myohemoglobinuric acute renal failure) for many years, and (d) a new diagnostic procedure, a computed tomography (CT) scan, had been developed and could be employed.

This disorder has gradually been recognized internationally during the past 26 years. It is quoted in the section on "Renal Hypouricemia" in *UpToDate* (electronic clinical reference on line). In Korea, several studies reported this disorder as patchy renal vasoconstriction [129]. Furthermore, the weekly magazine *Shukan Bunshun* (September 16, 2004) enlightened Japanese people about this disorder. On April 8, 2005, I gave a lecture entitled "Educational Lecture 9: Exercise-Induced Acute Renal Failure" at the 102nd general meeting of the Japanese Society of Internal Medicine [162].

The following issues, including the etiology, remain to be clarified: (a) the pathogenesis of ALPE, (b) the prevention of relapse, and future exercise guidance, (c) why delayed CT shows patchy contrast enhancement even in the recovery phase, (d) whether or not patchy renal vasoconstriction persists for 1–2 weeks, (e) why a contrast medium is present in the kidney for 72 h maximum, (f) the association between ALPE and disorders of type II muscle fibers, (g) the reasons for the less marked increases in serum myoglobin and creatine phosphokinase (CPK), and (h) why ALPE frequently develops in patients with renal hypouricemia.

These issues must be clarified in the future.

Acknowledgments

We thank the late Prof. Takeuchi, the late Dr. Berman, Prof. Hollenberg, the late Dr. Shinoda, staff in the Department of Nephrology, Kanazawa Medical University, and physicians in Keiju General Hospital and Asanogawa General Hospital for their cooperation.

Brief History of the Author

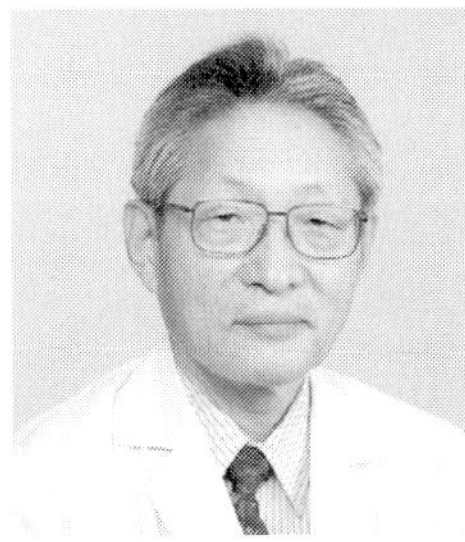

1965: Graduated from Kanazawa University School of Medicine.

1970: Completed a course in the Department of Medical Research, Kanazawa University Graduate School (First Department of Internal Medicine, instructed by Prof. Takeuchi), and obtained a doctorate of medicine (PhD).

1972–1973: Joined kidney disease study activities as a fellow at Mt. Sinai Hospital of Cleveland in the United States.

1973–1975: Studied under Prof. Hollenberg and Prof. Merrill at Peter Bent Brigham (the present Brigham and Women's) Hospital (Boston) and the School of Medicine, Harvard University, in the United States.

1975: After returning to Japan, took office as an associate professor in the Department of Nephrology, Kanazawa Medical University.

April 1989: Took office as a professor in the Department of Nephrology, Kanazawa Medical University, and as a professor at the General Medical Research Institute.

September 1994: Took office as the chief professor in the Department of Nephrology, Kanazawa Medical University.

April 2004: After a departmental reorganization, took office as a professor in the Department of Kidney Function Therapeutics (Nephrology), Kanazawa Medical University.

March 2006: Retired at the normal retirement age.

April 2006: Emeritus Professor of Kanazawa Medical University and Department of Nephrology, Asanogawa General Hospital.

References

1. Ishikawa I, Saito Y, Shinoda A, Onouchi Z (1981) Evidence for patchy renal vasoconstriction in man: observation by CT scan. Nephron 27:31–34
2. Ishikawa I, Onouchi Z, Yuri T, Saito Y, Shinoda A, Yamamoto I (1982) Acute renal failure with severe loin pain and patchy renal vasoconstriction. In: Eliahou HE (ed) Acute renal failure. John Libbey, London, pp 224–229
3. Ishikawa I, Sakurai Y, Masuzaki S, Sugishita N, Shinoda A, Shikura N (1990) Exercise-induced acute renal failure in 3 patients with renal hypouricemia. Nippon Jinzo Gakkai Shi (Jpn J Nephrol) 32:923–928
4. Ishikawa I (2002) Acute renal failure with severe loin pain and patchy renal ischemia after anaerobic exercise in patients with or without renal hypouricemia. Nephron 91:559–570
5. Meyer-Betz F (1910) Beobachtugen an einem eigenartigen mit muskellahmungen verbundenen Fall von Hamoglobinurie. Dtsch Arch Klin Med 101:85–127
6. Howenstine JA (1960) Exertion-induced myoglobinuria and hemoglobinuria: simulation of acute glomerulonephritis. JAMA 173:493–499
7. Jackson RC (1970) Exercise-induced renal failure and muscle damage. Proc R Soc Med 63:566–570
8. Hamilton RW, Gardner LB, Penn AS, Goldberg M (1972) Acute tubular necrosis caused by exercise-induced myoglobinuria. Ann Intern Med 77:77–82
9. Knochel JP (1972) Exertional rhabdomyolysis. N Engl J Med 287:927–929
10. Matsumoto T, Terukina S, Yamaguchi T, Nagase M, Suzuki H, Oda T (1976) A case of acute renal failure caused by exertional myoglobinuria (in Japanese). J Jpn Soc Intern Med 65:920–926
11. Sayers SP, Clarkson PM (2002) Exercise-induced rhabdomyolysis. Curr Sports Med Rep 1:59–60
12. Knochel JP (1990) Catastrophic medical events with exhaustive exercise: "white collar rhabdomyolysis". Kidney Int 38:709–719
13. Ishikawa I, Onouchi Z, Saito Y, Kitada H, Shinoda A, Ushitani K, Tabuchi M, Suzuki M (1981) Renal cortex visualization and analysis of dynamic CT curves of the kidney. J Comput Assist Tomogr 5:695–701
14. Ishikawa I (1982) The nephrogram in acute renal failure. Invest Radiol 17:194
15. Pazmino P, Pyatt R, Williams E, Bohan L (1983) Computed tomography in renal ischemia. J Comput Assist Tomogr 7:102–105
16. Mangano FA, Zaontz M, Pahira JJ, Clark LR, Jaffe MH, Choyke PL, Zeman RK (1985) Computed tomography of acute renal failure secondary to rhabdomyolysis. J Comput Assist Tomogr 9:777–779
17. Braedel HU, Schindler E, Cullen P, Hoene E (1987) Demonstration of residual contrast medium in renal parenchyma using computerized tomography. J Urol 137:11–14

18. Lim TH, Lee JS, Choi BI, Kim IO, Suh CH, Han MC, Kim CW (1987) An explanation of renal hemodynamics in acute renal failure based on sequential CT in patients with Korean hemorrhagic fever. J Comput Assist Tomogr 11:474–479
19. Grainger RG (1972) Renal toxicity of radiological contrast media. Br Med Bull 28:191–195
20. Hennessy WT, Pollack HM, Banner MP, Wein AJ (1981) Radiologic evaluation of anuric patient: systematized approach. Urology 18:435–445
21. Ludmer LM, Chandeysson P, Barth WF (1993) Diphosphonate bone scan in an unusual case of rhabdomyolysis: a report and literature review. J Rheumatol 20:382–384
22. Ishikawa I, Ishii H, Saito T, Yuri T, Shinoda A, Urashima S (1987) Increased patchy renal accumulation of ^{99m}Tc-methylene diphosphonate in a patient with severe loin pain after exercise. Nephron 47:29–31
23. Ueda T, Ootani M, Kataoka K, Hayashi T (1979) Two cases of exercise-induced acute renal failure (in Japanese). Jin-To-Tohseki (Kidney Dial) 6:495–498
24. Ishikawa I (1981) Loin pain and acute renal failure after exercise at athletic meetings (in Japanese). Igaku-No-Ayumi (J Clin Exp Med) 119:920
25. Nishimura M, Takahara K (1985) A case of abnormal urinalysis found by a school health check-up with exercise-induced acute renal failure (Japanese abstract). Nippon Jinzo Gakkai Shi (Jpn J Nephrol) 27:1730
26. Ishii H, Ishikawa I, Saito T, Yuri T, Shinoda A, Urashima S (1987) Exercise-induced acute renal failure with patchy RI accumulation by bone-seeking scan (Japanese abstract). Nippon Jinzo Gakkai Shi (Jpn J Nephrol) 29:1551
27. Nakamura I, Fujimoto Y, Kohno S, Tsuyuki M, Okada M, Tsuzuki K, Ito S, Watanabe T (1992) A case of exercise-induced acute renal failure syndrome (in Japanese). Shonika-Shinryo (J Pediatr Pract) 55:1721–1724
28. Erley CM, Hirschberg RR, Hoefer W, Schaefer K (1989) Acute renal failure due to uric acid nephropathy in a patient with renal hypouricemia. Klin Wochenschr 67:308–312
29. Ozono Y, Harada T, Ogawa K, Kanamoto Y, Hara K (1994) Acute tubular necrosis with loin pain and persistent multiple wedge-shaped contrast enhancement on CT. Intern Med (Tokyo) 33:53–55
30. Yoshiya K, Yoshikawa N, Ito S, Nakanishi K, Shimomura M, Iijima I, Nakamura H (1995) Exercise-induced acute renal failure in three patients with hypouricemia (in Japanese). Jin-To-Tohseki (Kidney Dial) 38:435–438
31. Ooi K, Ichida K, Okabe H, Kato N, Nakamura K, Kubo H, Kawamura T, Hosoya T, Jyou K (1998) A case of renal hypouricemia with exercise-induced acute renal failure (in Japanese). J Jpn Soc Intern Med 87:732
32. Kuroki Y, Shinozaki M, Higashi H (2002) A case with rhabdomyolysis and renal hypouricemia after exercise-induced acute renal failure (Japanese abstract). Nippon Jinzo Gakkai Shi (Jpn J Nephrol) 44:539
33. Kanegae K, Anai H, Kabajima K, Takemasa K, Nakajima Y, Seijima A, Tamura M (2003) A case of renal hypouricemia with acute renal failure after exercise (Japanese abstract). Rinsho-To-Kenkyu (Jpn J Clin Exp Med) 80:1346–1347
34. Sato T, Kuno T, Tashiro K, Fujita I, Miyazaki S (1998) Exercise-induced acute renal failure in a girl with renal hypouricemia. Acta Paediatr Jpn 40:93–95
35. Ishikawa I, Masuzaki S, Saito T, Yuri T, Shinoda A, Tsujigiwa M (1989) Magnetic resonance imaging in renal infarction and ischemia. Nephron 51:99–102
36. Ishikawa I, Nakagawa M, Hayama S, Yoshida S, Date T (2005) Acute renal failure with severe loin pain and patchy renal ischaemia after anaerobic exercise (ALPE) (exercise-induced acute renal failure) in a father and child with URAT1 mutations beyond the W258X mutation. Nephrol Dial Transplant 20:1015

37. Kumano K, Mashimo S, Sakai T (1980) Three cases of acute renal failure induced by untrained exercise (Japanese abstract). Nippon Jinzo Gakkai Shi (Jpn J Nephrol) 22:1579
38. Rikitake O, Nishihara S, Tashio N, Nakashima Y, Naito S, Arakawa K, Takebayashi S (1983) Two cases of exercise-induced acute renal failure (Japanese abstract). Naika (Intern Med) 51:759–762
39. Kuhn K, Wiemeyer A, Gause A, Helmchen U, Koch KM, Eisenbach GM (1984) Non-hyoglobinuric acute renal failure (ARF) after intensive muscular exercise and intake of analgesics. Kidney Int 25:170
40. Yamagata Y, Koga N (1984) A case of acute renal failure with severe loin pain and patchy wedge-shaped contrast enhancement after exercise due to renal artery spasm (Japanese abstract). Nippon Jinzo Gakkai Shi (Jpn J Nephrol) 26:1682–1683
41. Ishikawa I, Tateishi K, Onouchi Z, Saito Y, Futyu Y, Shinoda A, Yuri T (1985) Persistent wedge-shaped contrast enhancement of the kidney. Urol Radiol 7:45–47
42. Matsuura M, Kaneman K, Hanai J (1986) Two cases of acute renal failure with loin pain and nausea after exercise, revealing swelling of medullary pyramid on ultrasonography (Japanese abstract). Nippon Jinzo Gakkai Shi (Jpn J Nephrol) 28:1663
43. Hotta O, Taguma Y, Suzuki K, Futagi G, Kurosawa T, Takahashi H, Ishizaki M, Son T, Nakamichi G (1987) Four cases of acute renal failure mainly due to renal vasoconstriction (Japanese abstract). Nippon Jinzo Gakkai Shi (Jpn J Nephrol) 29:1489
44. Murakami T, Itagaki A, Takahashi H (1988–1989) A change of urinary proteins from a glomerular pattern to a tubular pattern during a late diuretic phase of acute renal failure. Child Nephrol Urol 9:160–162
45. Sakurauchi Y, Tsuyuki M, Okazaki Y, Sugiyama T, Yamamoto T (1990) Acute renal failure in the patient with hypouricemia (in Japanese). Jin-To-Tohseki (Kidney Dial) 29:845–848
46. Han JS, Kim YG, Kim S, Lee MC, Lee JS, Kim SH (1991) Bone scintigraphy in acute renal failure with severe loin pain and patchy renal vasoconstriction. Nephron 59:254–260
47. Kim SH, Han MC, Han JS, Kim S, Lee JS (1991) Exercise-induced acute renal failure and patchy renal vasoconstriction: CT and MR findings. J Comput Assist Tomogr 15:985–988
48. Numabe A, Tsukada H, Sugimoto T, Ono H, Hirao S, Abe M, Yagi S (1992) A case of acute renal failure in a patient with idiopathic hypouricemia (in Japanese with English abstract). Nippon Jinzo Gakkai Shi (Jpn J Nephrol) 34:841–845
49. Igarashi T, Sekine T, Sugimura H, Hayakawa H, Arayama T (1993) Acute renal failure after exercise in a child with renal hypouricaemia. Pediatr Nephrol 7:292–293
50. Kihara M, Ikeda Y, Shibata K, Masumori S, Ikegami T, Kitamura H, Ebira H (1993) Acute renal failure after a mild physical exercise in idiopathic renal hypouricaemia. Nephrol Dial Transplant 8:1384–1386
51. Shoji T, Hayashi T, Kitamura E, Okada N, Nakanishi I, Tsubakihara Y, Fushimi H, Kotoh K (1993) Clinico-pathological features in exercise-induced acute renal failure (in Japanese). Med J Osaka Pref 16:57–61
52. Hisanaga S, Kawamura M, Uchida T, Kondho H, Yoshida T (1994) Exercise-induced renal failure in a patient with hyperuricosuric hypouricemia. Nephron 66:475–476
53. Watanabe N, Shimizu M, Kageyama M, Kamei T, Seto H, Kakishita M (1994) Diffuse increased renal uptake on bone scintigraphy in acute tubular necrosis. Clin Nuc Med 19:19–21
54. Yoshie M, Tamura Y, Iijima Y, Nagata A, Kato M, Shigematsu S (1994) A case of non-oliguric acute renal failure after exercise (in Japanese). Shinshu Renal Seminar 1:87–90

55. Hiraishi K, Ohmori M, Murao S, Yamaguchi M (1994) A case of exercise-induced acute renal failure (in Japanese with English abstract). Jpn J Clin Urol 48:145–147
56. Hartman DS, Hopper KD (1994) Genitourinary case of the day. Exercise-induced acute renal failure. Am J Roentgenol 162:1452–1453
57. Fujieda M, Yokoyama W, Oishi N, Okada T, Kurashige T, Hamada G (1995) Acute renal failure after exercise in a child with renal hypouricemia. Acta Paediatr Jpn 37:642–644
58. Sanders LR (1995) Exercise-induced acute renal failure associated with ibuprofen, hydrochlorothiazide, and triamterene. J Am Soc Nephrol 5:2020–2023
59. Yeun JY, Hasbargen JA (1995) Renal hypouricemia: prevention of exercise-induced acute renal failure and a review of the literature. Am J Kidney Dis 25:937–946
60. Nagata T, Umeda Y, Tajima K, Inada M (1995) A case of idiopathic hypouricemia with acute renal failure after exercise (Japanese abstract). Nippon Jinzo Gakkai Shi (Jpn J Nephrol) 37:750
61. Tsunei T, Taguma Y, Sudou K, Horikago I, Hotta O, Chiba S, Miyazawa S, Oda T (1995) Seven cases with renal hypouricemia, complicated with acute renal failure after mild exercise (Japanese abstract). Nippon Jinzo Gakkai Shi (Jpn J Nephrol) 37:692
62. Ninomiya M, Ito Y, Nishi A, Matsumoto T, Koga A, Hori Y, Nishida H, Nomura G, Kato H (1996) Recurrent exercise-induced acute renal failure in renal hypouricemia. Acta Paediatr 85:1009–1011
63. Sakemi T, Ikeda Y, Matsuo Y, Kudo S, Nishihara G, Baba N (1996) Renal wedge-shaped lesions on computed tomography and ultrasonography in two patients who developed acute renal failure with severe loin pain after exercise. Nephron 73:679–681
64. Hirade S, Yasumoto K, Ueno H, Kyoda F, Izumino K, Takada M, Inoue H (1996) Three cases of acute renal failure with loin pain after exercise. J Jpn Soc Intern Med 85:642
65. Katano K, Koni I, Konoshita T, Kawano M, Okamoto H, Mabuchi H (1996) Sibling cases of renal hypouricemia with exercise-induced acute renal failure (Japanese abstract). Jpn J Dial Ther 29:883
66. Tazawa M, Morooka M, Takeichi S, Minowa S, Yasaki T (1996) Exercise-induced acute renal failure observed in a boy with idiopathic renal hypouricemia caused by postsecretory reabsorption defect of uric acid (in Japanese with English abstract). Nippon Jinzo Gakkai Shi (Jpn J Nephrol) 38:407–412
67. Momose A, Kudou D, Nishimura S, Sawada Y, Kitagawa M, Funao T, Suzuki Y (1996) A case of exercise-induced acute renal failure due to uric acid nephropathy in patient with cystinuria (in Japanese). Jin-To-Tohseki (Kidney Dial) 41:853–857
68. Izumi M, Yokoyama K, Yamauchi A, Horio M, Imai E (1997) A young man with acute renal failure and severe loin pain. Nephron 76:215–217
69. Ueda O, Oka T, Kyan H (1997) A case of renal hypouricemia with exercise-induced acute renal failure and cerebral infarction (in Japanese with English abstract). J Jpn Pediatr Soc 101:1620–1625
70. Watanabe M, Ishikawa I, Saigan T, Kimura S, Sakamoto K, Yamaya H, Nakamura M, Sakamoto S, Asaka M, Tomosugi N, Yuri T, Nakazawa T, Saito Y (1997) Exercise-induced acute renal failure with severe loin pain in two ADPKD patients (Japanese abstract). Nippon Jinzo Gakkai Shi (Jpn J Nephrol) 39:95
71. Numabe A, Teranishi M, Katagiri M, Futoo Y, Ono F, Ogawa Y, Abe M, Matsuoka H (1997) Two cases of hereditary renal hypouricemia complicated with exercise-induced acute renal failure (Japanese abstract). Nippon Jinzo Gakkai Shi (Jpn J Nephrol) 39:56
72. Sakuda T, Uehara G (1997) A case of renal hypouricemia with acute renal failure after exercise (Japanese abstract). Nippon Jinzo Gakkai Shi (Jpn J Nephrol) 39:577
73. Nagasawa Y, Tanaka A, Nakamura H, Fujita Y, Tanaka Z, Fujii M, Kobayashi A (1997) A case of exercise-induced ARF whose renal blood flow was observed by the

Doppler method (Japanese abstract). Nippon Jinzo Gakkai Shi (Jpn J Nephrol) 39:576

74. Yim JJ, Oh KH, Chin H, Ahn C, Kim SH, Han JS, Kim S, Lee JS (1998) Exercise-induced acute renal failure in a patient with congenital renal hypouricaemia. Nephrol Dial Transplant 13:994–997
75. Ueda N, Tanaka Y, Hyoudou S, Hamamoto K, Nishi Y (1998) A case of exercise-induced acute renal failure due to renal hypouricemia (in Japanese). Shonika-Rinsho (Jpn J Pediatr) 51:401–404
76. Itami N, Ohira S, Koga Y (1998) A case of renal hypouricemia with acute renal failure-uric acid changes by treadmill test (in Japanese). J Jpn Soc Pediatr Nephrol 18:51–53
77. Hisanaga S, Ueno N, Inagaki H, Tokura T, Uezono S, Yokota N, Fujimoto S, Eto T (1999) Exercise-induced acute renal failure associated with renal vasoconstriction (in Japanese with English abstract). Nippon Jinzo Gakkai Shi (Jpn J Nephrol) 41:406–412
78. Shimizu T, Kure M (1998) A case of exercise-induced acute renal failure probably due to renal vasoconstriction (Japanese abstract). Nippon Jinzo Gakkai Shi (Jpn J Nephrol) 40:493
79. Morita H, Okamoto K, Kohno K, Nishida H, Koga A, Wada Y, Usui M, Ueda S, Okuda M (1998) A recurrent case of acute renal failure after abrupt intense exercise (Japanese abstract). Nippon Jinzo Gakkai Shi (Jpn J Nephrol) 40:425
80. Kumabe T, Nishimura H, Uchida M, Kojima K, Ogho Y, Terasaki H, Hayabuchi N, Koga A, Nishida H, Hayashi H (1998) Two cases of exercise-induced acute renal failure (in Japanese). Rinsho Gazou (Clinical Imaging) 14:1426–1431
81. Oshima S, Abe S (1998) Exercise-induced acute renal failure in an infantryman with idiopathic renal hypouricemia (in Japanese with English abstract). National Defense Med J 45:273–278
82. Yokota K, Hirata K, Onbe T (1999) A case of exercise-induced acute renal failure without renal hypouricemia (Japanese abstract). Ehime Igaku 18:119
83. Tsubakihara Y, Susuki A, Togawa M, Hayashi K, Syouji T, Okada M, Izumi M, Imai E (1999) A case of renal dysfunction with severe loin pain after intensive exercise (in Japanese). Jpn J Clin Dial (Tokyo) 15:1313–1320
84. Ueda K, Takeuchi H, Takeuchi M, Kinoshita O, Katoh H (1999) A case of acute renal failure induced by exercise (Japanese abstract). Jpn J Dial Ther 32:770
85. Onbe T, Yokota K, Hirata K (1999) A case of exercise-induced acute renal failure without renal hypouricemia and without history of intake of NSAID (Japanese abstract). Jpn J Dial Ther 32:770
86. Miyata J (1999) A case with renal hypouricemia complicated with exercise-induced acute renal failure alleviated by ACE inhibitor (in Japanese). Miyazaki Igaku Gakkai Shi 23:162–166
87. Hasegawa M, Kawashima S, Toba T, Shikano M, Hasegawa H, Tomita M, Koide S, Asano S, Murakami K, Kato R (1999) Acute renal failure after exercise in a patient with renal hypouricemia. Clin Exp Nephrol 3:54–58
88. Kurihara I, Soma J, Sato H, Ikarashi T, Tsunoda K, Miura R, Suzuki T, Sato M, Furuyama T, Ito S, Saito T (2000) A case of exercise-induced acute renal failure in a patient with enhanced renal hypouricaemia. Nephrol Dial Transplant 15: 104–106
89. Kikuchi Y, Koga H, Yasutomo Y, Kawabata Y, Shimizu E, Naruse M, Kiyama S, Nonoguchi H, Tomita K, Sasatomi Y, Takebayashi S (2000) Patients with renal hypouricemia with exercise-induced acute renal failure and chronic renal dysfunction. Clin Nephrol 53:467–472
90. Watanabe T, Abe T, Oda Y (2000) Exercise-induced acute renal failure in a patient with renal hypouricemia. Pediatr Nephrol 14:851–852

91. Takayama K, Kawai H, Nabeshima K (2000) Three suspected cases of exercise-induced acute renal failure (Japanese abstract). Nippon Jinzo Gakkai Shi (Jpn J Nephrol) 42:442
92. Fujii T, Hasegawa S, Iesato K (2000) Two cases of exercise-induced acute renal failure—acute renal failure related to serum uric acid level (Japanese abstract). Nippon Jinzo Gakkai Shi (Jpn J Nephrol) 42:536
93. Ando R, Dohi M, Amano H, Yamauchi K, Senda Y, Ida T, Kubo A (2000) A case of exercise-induced acute renal failure: his clinical course followed by contrast enhanced color Doppler (Japanese abstract). Nippon Jinzo Gakkai Shi (Jpn J Nephrol) 42:537
94. Sudo H, Tuji M, Unishi G (2000) Exercise-induced acute renal failure in a boy with renal hypouricemia (in Japanese with English abstract). J Jpn Soc Pediatr Nephrol 13:33–37
95. Takeda Y, Fujimoto T, Uyama H, Shiiki H, Yamano S, Kanauchi M, Yabuta M, Dohi K (2001) Two cases of exercise-induced acute renal failure with idiopathic renal hypouricemia (in Japanese with English abstract). Nippon Jinzo Gakkai Shi (Jpn J Nephrol) 43:384–388
96. Lee JY, Cho JT, Park YJ, Shin MH, Koo CH, Park TY, Kim JS, Han SS, Kang JH (1996) A case of acute renal failure with severe loin pain and patchy renal vasoconstriction after exercise (in Korean with English abstract). Korean J Med 50:840–845
97. Shin J, Lee E, Kwon Y, Lee J, Cho S, Park C, Lee D, Kim M-S, Pyo H-J (1997) Exercise-induced acute renal failure associated with nonsteroidal anti-inflammatory drugs: report of 2 cases (in Korean with English abstract). Korean J Nephrol 16:607–611
98. Watanabe T, Abe T, Oda Y (2000) Exercise-induced acute renal failure in a patient with renal hypouricemia. Pediatr Nephrol 14:851–852
99. Chang HH, Kim HJ, Lee JJ, Kim JH, Lee TW, Ihm CG, Kim MJ (2001) Exercise-induced acute renal failure in a patient with renal hypouricemia (in Korean with English abstract). Korean J Nephrol 20:714–718
100. Hiraoka K, Kotaki Y, Takamitsu Y (2001) A case of hypouricemia developed acute renal failure after exercise (in Japanese). Rinsho Tohseki (Jpn J Clin Dial) 17:1625–1630
101. Murakami H, Kitazawa E, Iwamoto T, Watanabe S, Takahashi M, Owada M, Harada K (2001) A boy with exercise-induced acute renal failure without hypouricemia (Japanese abstract). J Jpn Soc Pediatr Nephrol 14:130
102. Nishikawa K, Yamada H, Miura N, Aoki T, Yoh T, Sakuma M, Futenma A, Miyai H (2001) Exercise-induced acute renal failure in a patient with whole nephron reabsorption disturbance of uric acid (Japanese abstract). Nippon Jinzo Gakkai Shi (Jpn J Nephrol) 43:468
103. Sato Y, Fujimoto S, Hisanaga S, Kawasaki Y, Eto T, Miyata J (2001) Exercise-induced acute renal failure in a patient with renal hypouricemia (in Japanese). Tsufu-to-KakusanTaisha (Gout Nucleic Acid Metab) 25:164–169
104. Toyoura M, Mikami T, Tachikawa E, Nagabuchi H, Chikamoto Y, Watanabe M, Hattori M, Shiraga H, Ito K (2001) A case of renal hypouricemia with exercise-induced acute renal failure (Japanese abstract). Nippon Jinzo Gakkai Shi (Jpn J Nephrol) 43:534
105. Nomura T (2001) A case of exercise-induced acute renal failure with renal hypouricemia (Japanese abstract). J Jpn Soc Clin Internist 16:312
106. Yamazaki H, Ohkubo S, Suzuki T, Kasahara T, Kobayashi Y, Uchiyama H (2001) A case of exercise-induced acute renal failure without idiopathic renal hypouricemia (in Japanese). Jin-To-Tohseki (Kidney Dial) 51:407–411
107. Ohta T, Sakano T, Ogawa T, Kato J, Awaya Y, Kihara H, Kinoshita Y (2002) Exercise-induced acute renal failure with renal hypouricemia: a case report and a review of the literature. Clin Nephrol 58:313–316

108. Watanabe T (2002) Patchy renal vasoconstriction after exercise in a child without renal hypouricemia. Pediatr Nephrol 17:284–286
109. Choi SC, Kim YG, Do JH, Kim JA, Lee YK, Lee HH, Yoon SJ, Huh W, Kim DJ, Oh HY, Kim B (2002) Patient with renal hypouricemia and exercise-induced acute renal failure (in Korean with English abstract). Korean J Nephrol 21:312–316
110. Mikami H, Tazawa S, Fujiwara M, Saito M, Saito A, Abukawa D, Maeda H, Takahashi K (2002) A case of exercise-induced acute renal failure without renal hypouricemia (Japanese abstract). J Jpn Pediatr Soc 106:1489
111. Someya T, Hattori M, Toyoura M, Mikami T, Tachikawa E, Nagabuchi H, Chikamoto Y, Watanabe M, Shiraga H, Ito K (2002) Three children with idiopathic renal hypouricemia with acute renal failure after exercise (in Japanese). J Jpn Soc Pediatr Nephrol 22:123–125
112. Inagaki A, Abe K, Kawase Y, Itoh I (2002) Exercise-induced acute renal failure in a patient with renal hypouricemia (in Japanese). J Osaka Dial Ther 20:73–77
113. Yoneda Y, Wakisaka Y, Shimada H (2002) A case of renal hypouricemia with exercise-induced acute renal failure followed by recurrent renal dysfunction after strenuous exercise (Japanese abstract). Nippon Jinzo Gakkai Shi (Jpn J Nephrol) 44:315
114. Shinzato T, Kamohara R, Namie S, Tamaguchi K (2002) A case of exercise-induced acute renal failure with idiopathic renal hypouricemia (in Japanese with English abstract). Proc Sasebo City General Hosp 28:69–71
115. Shimamine R, Miyake C, Muratani Y, Miyazaki M, Kouno S, Harada T, Taguchi N (2002) The cases of exercise-induced acute renal failure in siblings with idiopathic renal hypouricemia (in Japanese). Jin-To-Tohseki (Kidney Dial) 52:235–238
116. Numabe A, Hishinuma A, Ishimitu T, Matuoka H, Ieiri A (2002) A case of idiopathic renal hypouricemia with exercise-induced acute renal failure (Japanese abstract). J Jpn Soc Endocrinol 78:178
117. Tanaka M, Itoh K, Matsushita K, Matsushita K, Wakita N, Adachi M, Nonoguchi H, Kitamura K, Hosoyamada M, Endou H, Tomita K (2003) Two male siblings with hereditary renal hypouricemia and exercise-induced ARF. Am J Kidney Dis 42:1287–1292
118. Hatsukano M, Takeuchi H, Katsube Y, Fujita T, Matsuoka K, Tsuchiya M (2003) A case of exercise-induced acute renal failure with renal hypouricemia (Japanese abstract). J Nippon Med Sch 70:585
119. Koyama M, Ishii M, Watanabe K (2003) A case of exercise-induced acute renal failure and patchy renal vasoconstriction (Japanese abstract). J Jpn Radiol Soc 63:S413
120. Sehara Y, Nagake Y, Toda N, Nakamura A, Hiramatsu M, Nose S (2003) Exercise-induced acute renal failure with hypouricemia: a case report (in Japanese with English abstract). J Okayama Saiseikai General Hospital 35:24–28
121. Ohkuma T, Minagawa T, Takada N, Oono M, Oda H, Ohashi H (2003) A case of renal hypouricemia with exercise-induced acute renal failure (Japanese abstract). Nippon Jinzo Gakkai Shi (Jpn J Nephrol) 45:647
122. Tsuruta M, Hattori K, Miura Y, Furuse A, Kohno T, Nakasato H, Karashima S, Hattori S (2003) Exercise-induced acute renal failure in two boys with renal hypouricemia (Japanese abstract). J Jpn Soc Pediatr Nephrol 16:165
123. Inoue H, Imamura S, Toyota A, Amemiya M, Tabei K (2004) A case of vasoconstrictive nephropathy (Japanese abstract). Nippon Jinzo Gakkai Shi (Jpn J Nephrol) 46:626
124. Kinjyo K, Miyagi M, Yamashiro M (2004) A case of acute renal failure due to renal hypouricemia (Japanese abstract). J Okinawa Med Assoc 43:94
125. Takada H, Tsuchida Y, Nishimura S, Hara I (2004) A case of acute renal failure developed after exercise. J Jpn Soc Dial Ther 37:1829
126. Nagaba Y, Sano T, Takeuchi Y, Moriya T, Saruta T, Hamura M, Sakamoto N, Higashihara M, Kamata K (2004) A case of renal hypouricemia with recurrent

exercise-induced acute renal failure (Japanese abstract). Nippon Jinzo Gakkai Shi (Jpn J Nephrol) 46:609

127. Park HJ, Kim MJ, Jin DK, Cheong HI, Choi Y, Ko KW, Park JM, Yeun KM (1991) Acute renal failure with back pain after exercise (in Korean with English abstract). J Korean Pediatr Soc 34:863–868
128. Aoki T, Ishida T, Sasaki T, Masuko Y, Ishida M, Tateshita K, Sakurai T, Uede T (2004) A case of renal hypouricemia with exercise-induced acute renal failure (Japanese abstract). Presented at the 233rd Hokkaido Regional Meeting of the Japanese Society of Internal Medicine
129. Shin YM, Han HS, Goo JC, Park SS, Lim SW, Kim M-O, Kwon SK, Kim H-Y, Han GS (2005) Clinical manifestations of acute renal failure with loin pain developed after anaerobic exercise (in Korean with English abstract). Korean J Nephrol 24:64–70
130. Nishida H, Kaida H, Ishibashi M, Baba K, Kouno K, Okuda S (2005) Evaluation of exercise-induced acute renal failure in renal hypouricemia using Tc-99m DTPA renography. Ann Nucl Med 19:325–329
131. Cheong HI, Kang JH, Lee JH, Ha IS, Kim S, Komoda F, Sekine T, Igarashi T, Choi Y (2005) Mutational analysis of idiopathic renal hypouricemia in Korea. Pediatr Nephrol 20:886–890
132. Hirashio H, Maki K, Naito T, Yorioka T (2005) A case of familial renal hypouricemia with acute renal failure after exercise (Japanese abstract). Nippon Jinzo Gakkai Shi (Jpn J Nephrol) 47:638
133. Terami T, Ohta Y, Sarai T, Hida K, Takeyama T, Ohishi T, Sato T, Yamadori I (2005) A case of renal hypouricemia with acute renal failure after exercise (Japanese abstract). Presented at the 92nd Chyugoku Regional Meeting of the Japanese Society of Internal Medicine
134. Yoshida M, Yagi N, Miyazato H, Sakuda A, Sunagawa H, Uehara G (2005) A case of hypouricemia of unknown etiology with exercise-induced acute renal failure (Japanese abstract). J Okinawa Med Assoc 44:129
135. Mori Y, Matsuo T, Tajima M, Okado T, Tsukamoto Y, Sasaki S (2005) Twin case of renal hypouricemia with exercise-induced acute renal failure (Japanese abstract). Nippon Jinzo Gakkai Shi (Jpn J Nephrol) 47:742
136. Fukuoka A, Maejima Y, Asada M, Kikumoto Y, Nakamura Y, Sugiyama S, Yamazaki Y, Makino H (2005) A case of idiopathic renal hypouricemia with exercise-induced acute renal failure (Japanese abstract). Presented at the 92nd Chyugoku Regional Meeting of the Japanese Society of Internal Medicine
137. Gabow PA, Kaehny WD, Kelleher SP (1982) The spectrum of rhabdomyolysis. Medicine (Baltimore) 61:141–152
138. Hasegawa M, Kawashima S, Toba T, Shikano M, Hasegawa H, Tomita M, Koide S, Asano S, Murakami K, Kato R (1999) Acute renal failure after exercise in a patient with hypouricemia. Clin Exp Nephrol 1:54–58
139. Ishii H, Ishikawa I, Masuzaki S, Sugishita N, Tateishi K, Kitada H, Yuri T, Shinode A (1989) A case of exercise-induced acute renal failure developed during the remission of minimal change nephrotic syndrome (Japanese abstract). Nippon Jinzo Gakkai Shi (Jpn J Nephrol) 30:1326–1327
140. Ishikawa I, Watanabe M, Saigan T, Nakazawa T, Tomosugi N, Yuri T, Saito Y (1997) Exercise-induced acute renal failure with severe loin pain in ADPKD patients. Acute renal failure—Towards 2000 (ISN Satellite Symposium), Cairns, Australia, 1997, p 87
141. Brumback RA, Feeback DL, Leech RW (1992) Rhabdomyolysis in childhood. A primer on normal muscle function and selected metabolic myopathies characterized by disordered energy production. Pediatr Clin North Am 39:821–858
142. Yamamoto M, Ito H (1997) Aerobic and anaerobic exercises (in Japanese). Clin Sport Med (Tokyo) 14:187–192

143. Koutsuki M, Yoshida T (1998) Anaerobic and aerobic exercises (in Japanese). Seikeigeka Kango (Orthop Nurs) 3:530–535
144. Armstrong RB, Warren GL, Warren JA (1991) Mechanisms of exercise-induced muscle fibre injury. Sports Med 12:184–207
145. Visweswaran P, Guntupalli J (1999) Rhabdomyolysis. Crit Care Clin 15:415–428
146. Little PJ, Sloper JS, de Wardener HE (1967) A syndrome of loin pain and haematuria associated with disease of peripheral renal arteries. Q J Med 36:253–259
147. Burden RP, Booth LJ, Ockenden BG, Boyd WN, Higgins PM, Aber GM (1975) Intrarenal vascular changes in adult patients with recurrent haematuria and loin pain: a clinical, histological and angiographic study. Q J Med 44:433–447
148. Fletcher P, Al-Khader AA, Parsons V, Aber GM (1979) The pathology of intrarenal vascular lesions associated with the loin-pain-haematuria syndrome. Nephron 24:150–154
149. Enomoto A, Kimura H, Chairoungdua A, Shigeta Y, Jutabha P, Cha SH, Hosoyamada M, Takeda M, Sekine T, Igarashi T, Matsuo H, Kikuchi Y, Oda T, Ichida K, Hosoya T, Shimokata K, Niwa T, Kanai Y, Endou H (2002) Molecular identification of a renal urate anion exchanger that regulates blood urate levels. Nature 417:447–452
150. Hisatome I, Ogino K, Kotake H, Ishiko R, Saito M, Hasegawa J, Mashiba H, Nakamoto S (1989) Cause of resistent hypouricemia in outpatients. Nephron 51:13–16
151. Igarashi T (1993) Normal serum uric acid concentrations for age and sex and incidence of renal hypouricaemia in Japanese school children. Pediatr Nephrol 7:239–240
152. Ames BN, Cathcart R, Schwiers E, Hochstein P (1981) Uric acid provides an antioxidant defense in humans against oxidant- and radical-caused aging and cancer: a hypothesis. Proc Natl Acad Sci USA 78:6858–6862
153. Murakami T, Kawakami H, Fukuda M, Furukawa S (1995) Patients with renal hypouricemia are prone to develop acute renal failure—why? Clin Nephrol 43:207–208
154. Perlstein TS, Gumieniak O, Hopkins PN, Murphey LJ, Brown NJ, Williams GH, Hollenberg NK, Fisher ND (2004) Uric acid and the state of the intrarenal renin–angiotensin system in humans. Kidney Int 66:1465–1470
155. Ichida K, Hosoyamada M, Hisatome I, Enomoto A, Hikita M, Endou H, Hosoya T (2004) Clinical and molecular analysis of patients with renal hypouricemia in Japan: influence of the URAT1 gene on urinary urate excretion. J Am Soc Nephrol 15:164–173
156. Paller MS, Hoidal JR, Ferris TF (1984) Oxygen free radicals in ischemic acute renal failure in the rat. J Clin Invest 74:1156–1164
157. Cooper CE, Vollaard NB, Choueiri T, Wilson MT (2002) Exercise, free radicals and oxidative stress. Biochem Soc Trans 30:280–285
158. Roberts LJ2nd, Morrow JD (1997) The generation and actions of isoprostanes. Biochim Biophys Acta 1345:121–135
159. Ishii H, Saitoh T, Ishikawa I (1997) Wedge-shaped enhancement on delayed CT scan during vasopressin infusion in rats (in Japanese with English abstract). J Kanazawa Med Univ 22:15–25
160. O'Regan S, Fong JS, Drummond KN (1979) Renal injury after muscle extract infusion in rats: absence of toxicity with myoglobin. Experientia 35:805–806
161. Blachar Y, Fong JS, de Chadarevian JP, Drummond KN (1981) Muscle extract infusion in rabbits. A new experimental model of the crush syndrome. Circ Res 49:114–124
162. Ishikawa I (2005) Exercise-induced acute renal failure (in Japanese). Nippon Naika Gakkai Zasshi (J Jpn Soc Intern Med) 94:1949–1955

Index